SIRTFOOD DIET

A Beginner's Guide To Weight Loss.

Activate Your Skinny Gene, Boost Metabolism, And Burn Fat.

|Including Tips To Prepare A Sirtfood Meal Plan.|

Table Of Contents

application, whether directly or indirectly, of any advice or information presented, whether for breach of contract, tort, negligence, personal injury, criminal intent, or under any other cause of action.

You agree to accept all risks of using the information presented inside this book.

You agree that by continuing to read this book, where appropriate and/or necessary, you shall consult a professional (including but not limited to your doctor, attorney, or financial advisor or such other advisor as needed) before using any of the suggested remedies, techniques, or information in this book.

INTRODUCTION

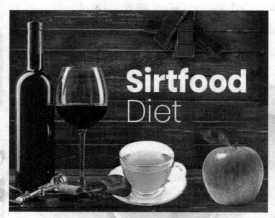

The Sirtfood diet continues to be a hot topic and involves people taking a diet rich in sirtfood. According to the founders of the diet, these special foods work by activating specific proteins called sirtuins in the body. Sirtuins are expected to protect the cells of the body against dying when under stress and regulate inflammation, metabolism, and aging. It is thought that sirtuins affect the ability of the body to burn fat and increase metabolism, leading to a loss of seven pounds of muscle per week. Some experts believe, however, that the loss of fat alone is unlikely, but instead reflects changes in glycogen stores in the skeletal muscle and the liver.

Even though diet encourages healthy foods, both your food and your daily calories are restrictive, especially in the initial stages. This also involves drinking water, which is higher than the existing daily recommendations in step one.

The second phase is known as the 14-day maintenance period, during which steady weight loss takes place. The authors believe that the loss of weight is sustainable and realistic. However, weight loss does not focus on the diet, and it's structured to consume the best foods that nature has to offer. They recommend eating three balanced, productive, sort food meals a day with one green sort of food juice for the long term.

We also should eat a mixture of various fruits and vegetables, not just those on the list

CHAPTER ONE: The Sirtfood Diet

New trendy diets appear regularly, and the Sirtfood Diet is among the most original.

This has become the favorite of famous European people and is popular for allowing chocolate and red wine.

Its creators stress that it is not a fad, but that the secret of freeing fat loss and preventing disease is the "sirtfoods."

Health professionals, however, warn that this diet may not be up to the hype and even be a bad idea.

This book provides a proven review of the Sirtfood Diet and its possible health benefits. What is the diet for sirtfood?
The Sirtfood Diet was developed by two famous nutritionists working at a private gym in the UK.

They publicize the diet as a new innovative nutritional and lifestyle plan that functions by activating your "skinny gene."

Sirtuins (SIRTs), a group of seven proteins present in the blood that has demonstrated the regulation of various functions, including inflammation, metabolism, and lifespan, are a foundation of this diet.

Some natural plant compounds can increase the body's protein level, and foods containing it have been referred to as "sirtfoods."

The Sirtfood Diet list of the "top sirtfoods" includes:

- Strawberries.

- Kale.

- Coffee.

- Red wine.

- Parsley.

- Onions.

- Extra virgin olive oil.

- Soy.

- Buckwheat.

- Dark chocolate (85% cocoa).

- Lovage.

- Red chicory.

- Turmeric.

- Matcha green tea.

- Walnuts.

- Arugula (rocket).

- Bird's eye chili.

- Blueberries.

- Medjool dates.

- Capers.

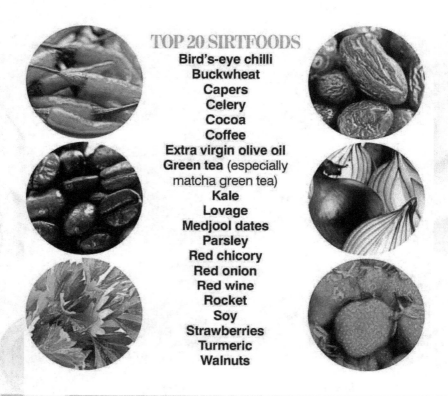

TOP 20 SIRTFOODS
Bird's-eye chilli
Buckwheat
Capers
Celery
Cocoa
Coffee
Extra virgin olive oil
Green tea (especially matcha green tea)
Kale
Lovage
Medjool dates
Parsley
Red chicory
Red onion
Red wine
Rocket
Soy
Strawberries
Turmeric
Walnuts

The diet combines sirtfoods with calorie constraints, both of which can cause the body to produce higher sirtuins.

The Sirtfood Diet book contains meals and recipes to follow, but many more Sirtfood Diet books are available.

The creators of the diet argue that after the sirtfood diet, you will lose weight rapidly while maintaining muscle mass and protecting yourself against chronic diseases.

When you have completed your diet, you are advised to keep your daily intake of sirtfoods and green juice on the menu.

Will it work?

The writers of the Sirtfood Diet make audacious claims, including that your diet can overload weight loss, enhance your "skinny gene" and prevent illness.
The problem is that there is not much evidence to support them.

There is no convincing evidence to date that the Sirtfood Diet has a more beneficial weight loss effect than any other calorie-controlled diet.

And although many of these foods are healthy, no long-term human trials have been conducted to determine if eating food that is rich in sirtfoods get health tangible benefits.

The Sirtfood Diet nevertheless describes the results of the pilot study carried out by the authors with the participation of 39 people from their fitness center. Nonetheless, it seems that the findings of this analysis were not published elsewhere.

The participants observed the diet for one week and exercised every day. They lost 7 pounds (3,2 kg) on average at the end of the week and keep or even gained muscle mass.

However, these findings are hardly surprising. Limiting your calorie consumption to 1,000 calories at the same time will almost always lead to weight loss.

Nevertheless, this form of rapid loss of weight is neither actual nor last long, and after a week they start, participants did not follow this study to see whether they had recovered any of the typical weight back.

When the body is depleted of nutrition, it uses its emergency energy reserves of glycogen, as well as fat and muscle.

Each glycogen molecule requires 3–4 water molecules to be stored. It also gets rid of this water when your body uses glycogen. It is referred to as "water weight."

Only about one-third of the weight loss in the first week of extreme calorie limitation is fat, and the other two-thirds are muscle, water, and glycogen.

As your calorie consumption increases, your body fills up its glycogen shops and weight returns immediately.

Sadly, this kind of calorie restriction will also decrease the body's metabolic rate, and you need even fewer calories a day for energy than before.

This diet will probably help you shed a few pounds at the start, but it will probably come back once your food is done.

Concerning disease prevention, three weeks seems to be probably insufficient to have a quantifiable long-term impact.

On the other hand, it might be a smart idea to add sirtfood to your daily diet on a long-term basis. Yet, in that case, you might also save the diet and now continue to do so.

Following the Sirtfood Diet

The Sirtfood Diet lasts three weeks and is divided into two phases. Then you can continue to 'sirtify' your diet with as many sirtfoods as possible.

The essential recipes for these two phases are contained in The Sirtfood Diet Book, published by the creators of the diet. You must buy it to follow the diet.

The foods are made of sirtfoods which contain the "top 20 sirtfoods" as well. Most ingredients and sirtfoods can be found easily.
The essential ingredients are matcha, lovage, green tea powder, buckwheat, and are expensive or difficult to find.

Much of the diet is a green juice, which you have to make between one and three times a day. A juicer (a blender doesn't work) and a kitchen scale are needed because the products are listed in weight. The following is the recipe:

Green Sirtfood Juice:

- 30 grams (rocket) (1 oz.)
- arugula.
- 75 grams kale (2.5 oz).
- 1 cm ginger (0.5 in).
- Five parsley grams.
- Two sticks celery.
- Half a teaspoon matcha green tea.
- Half a lemon.
- Half a green apple.

Juice and pour into a glass all ingredients except the powder of green tea and the lemon. Juice the lemon by hand and apply both the lemon juice and green tea powder.

Phase 1

The first process lasts seven days, with a drop in calories and plenty of green juice. It is intended to start your weight loss in seven days and claims to help lose 7 pounds (3.2 kg).

In Phase One, the calorie intake is limited to 1,000 calories for the first three days. You drink three green juices a day plus one meal. Every day, you can select from the recipes in the book that are primarily sirtfoods.

Misshapen tofu, the sirtfood omelet, or a shrimp stir-fry with buckwheat noodles are some of the meal examples.

Days 4–7 of Phase 1 you should increase the calorie intake to 1,500. It involves two green juices a day and another two sirtfoods that can be picked from the book.

Phase 2

The second process lasts two weeks. You should continue to lose weight during this "maintenance" phase.

In this phase, there is no specific calorie limit. Instead, you eat three sirtfood meals and a green juice a day once meals are taken from the book's recipes.

After the food

For more weight loss, you can repeat these two steps as much as you like.

However, after these stages, you are advised to continue to "sirtify" your diet by frequently including sirtfood in your meal.

There are several Sirtfood Diet books full of recipes. Sirtfoods can also be included in your diet as a snack or in your own recipes.

Therefore, every day you are advised to continue to drink green tea.

The Sirtfood Diet, therefore, becomes a lifestyle change rather than a one-time diet. Are new superfoods Sirtfoods?
Nobody denies that sirtfoods are right for you. They often contain high nutrients and plenty of healthy plant compounds.
Besides, studies have linked many of the foods recommended for the Sirtfood Diet to health benefits.

Eating moderate quantities of dark chocolate with a high cocoa content, for example, can lower the risk of heart disease and help combat inflammation.

Green tea will reduce the risk of stroke and diabetes and lower blood pressure.

And turmeric has anti-inflammatory characteristics that generally have beneficial effects on your body and can even protect against chronic inflammatory diseases.
In fact, most sirtfoods have shown health benefits in humans.

However, there is preliminary evidence of the health benefits of increasing sirtuin protein levels. Nonetheless, animal and cell line work has shown promising results.

Researchers have found, for example, that increased levels of specific sirtuin proteins result in a longer lifetime in yeast, worms, and mice.

And during the restriction of fasting or calories, sirtuin protein tells the body to burn more fat for energy and develop insulin sensitivity. A study found that increased sirtuin concentrations resulted in fat loss. There is evidence that sirtuins can also help reduce inflammatory diseases, inhibit tumor growth, and slow the development of heart disease and Alzheimer's disease.

While experiments in mice and human cell lines showed promising results, no social studies have investigated the effects of increasing sirtuin levels.

It is, therefore, unclear whether increased levels of sirtuin protein in the body result in a longer lifespan or a lower risk of cancer in humans.
Research is underway to develop compounds that increase the body's sirtuin levels effectively. In this way, human studies will continue to examine the human health effects of sirtuins.

Until then, the consequences of increased sirtuin levels cannot be determined.

Is it sound and sustainable?

Sirtfoods are almost every healthy choice, and their antioxidant or anti-inflammatory properties may even give some health benefits.

However, eating just a handful of especially healthy foods can not satisfy all nutritional needs of your body.

Sirtfood is unnecessary and does not provide simple, specific health benefits over any other diet.

Also, eating only 1,000 calories is usually not recommended without a physician's supervision. Even a daily consumption of 1,500 calories is too restrictive for many people.

The diet also requires up to three green juices a day to drink. While juices are a good source of vitamins and minerals, they also contain almost no healthy fiber as whole fruits and vegetables do. They are also a source of sugar.

Moreover, drinking juice all day long is a bad idea for both your blood sugar and teeth.

Not to mention that because the diet is so low in calories and food choice, vitamins, protein, and minerals are most likely deficient, particularly during the first phase.

This diet can be challenging to stick with for three weeks because of low-calorie levels and restrictive food choices.

In addition to the high initial costs of purchasing the juicer, books, and other rare and expensive ingredients and time-consuming meals and juices, this diet has become unfeasible and unsustainable for many.

Safety and effects on the side

Even if the first step of the Sirtfood Diet is low in calories and nutritionally incomplete, the average healthy adult does not have any real safety issues given the short duration of the diet.

But, calorie restriction and consuming juice most of the first few days of the diet can cause harmful changes in blood sugar levels for people with diabetes.

However, even a healthy person may suffer mainly from hunger and some other side effects.

Just 1,000-1,500 calories a day can leave almost everyone hungry, mainly if you just drink juice, which is low in fiber, a nutrient that will keep you full.

During phase one, due to calorie limitation, you may experience other side effects such as light heading, fatigue, and irritability.

It is unlikely to have serious health consequences for the otherwise healthy adult if the diet is followed for only three weeks.

The Sirtfood Diet is full of healthy foods but is not healthy.

Its theory and health claims are not to mention based on significant extrapolations from preliminary scientific evidence.
When you add sirtfoods to your diet, it's not a bad idea and can even offer health benefits, but your diet itself looks like a fad.

Save yourself the money and go for healthy, long-term food changes.

The science and the story of Sirtuins

Sirtuins help your cellular quality of life to be regulated. This is how it works, what they're doing to the body, and why depends on NAD+ to work.

Sirtuins are really a family of cellular health-regulating proteins, and they play a crucial role in cell homeostasis control. Homeostasis requires equilibrium of the cell. However, in the presence of nicotinamide adenine dinucleotide, NAD+, a coenzyme discovered in all living cells, sirtuins can function only.

How The Sirtuins regulate NAD+ cell health

Think of the cells in your body like an office. In the office, many people work on different tasks with the ultimate objective: remaining profitable and fulfilling the mission of the company as effectively as possible. There are many parts of cells that work on different tasks with the ultimate goal: stay healthy and work as long as possible. Just as company priorities change because of various internal and external factors, so are cell priorities. Somebody has to run the office and regulate what happens when, who will do it, and when to change course. That would be your CEO in the office. In the body, it's your sirtuins on the cellular level.

Sirtuins are the seven protein family that has a role to play in cellular health. Sirtuins can only act in the presence of NAD+, and the coenzyme presents in living cells, nicotinamide adenine dinucleotide. NAD+ is essential for the metabolism of cells and hundreds of other biological processes. If sirtuins are CEOs of business, NAD+ is the money spent by the CEO and the staff while maintaining lights and paying the rent on office space. Without it, business and the body cannot function. However, NAD+ levels decline with age and also restrict the role of sirtuins with age. It's not that easy, as all things and in the human body. Sirtuins control everything that takes place in your cells.

Sirtuins are proteins. What is that meaning?

Protein may sound like protein intake, as is present in beans and meats, and even in protein shakes, but in this case, we are thinking about protein molecules that act in different roles in the body's cells. Think of protein as a company's departments, each focusing on its own specific function and coordinating with other departments.

Hemoglobin, a well-known carbohydrate in the body, is part of the protein family of globins and the oxygen transport throughout the blood. Myoglobin is the counterpart of hemoglobin, and together they make up the globin family.

Your body has almost 60,000 protein families in many departments! And one of those families is sirtuins. While the hemoglobin is just one of a two-protein family, myoglobin is a group of seven.

Of seven sirtuins in the cell, three work in the mitochondria, three work in the nucleus, and one works in the cytoplasm, each with a range of roles. However, the fundamental function of sirtuins is to extract acetyl groups from other proteins.

Similar reactions are regulated by acetyl groups. These are physical protein tags that other proteins know and respond to. If proteins are the cell departments, and DNA is the CEO, each department head has an accessibility status of the acetyl groups. For instance, if a protein is available, the sirtuin can work with it in order to make something happen, just like the CEO may work with a department manager.

Sirtuins work with acetyl groups through deacetylation. This means that they know that a molecule contains an acetyl group and then eliminate the acetyl group that removes the molecule for its function. One way sirtuins function is to eliminate biological proteins such as histones from the acetyl groups (deacetylating).

Sirtuins, for example, deacetylate histones, proteins that are part of a compact type of DNA known as chromatin. The histone is an abundant voluminous protein that is wrapped in the DNA. Speak of it as a Christmas tree, and the DNA beach is the main beach. The chromatin is open or unwound, whether the histones are of an acetyl group.

This unwound chromatin means that the transcription of the DNA is necessary. However, it doesn't have to be left relaxed, as it is vulnerable to damage, just like the Christmas light, or the bulbs, whether they are unhandy or too long, can be harmed. The chromatin is blocked, or the gene expression is interrupted or silenced as the histones are deacetylated by air tubes.

For around 20 years, we have known only about sirtuins, and their primary feature was discovered in the 1990s.

Sirtuins' Discovery and History

In the 1970s, the first sirtuin, named SIR2, was discovered by geneticist Dr. Amar Klar to classify it as a gene regulating yeast cell mate ability. Years later, researchers found genes in the 1990s, that were identical in form to SIR2 in some species such as fruit flies, worms, and were then called sirtuins by these SIR2 counterparts. Each organism had different numbers of sirtuins. For instance, yeast has five sirtuins, one is bacterial, seven are mice, and seven are human.

The existence of sirtuins across species means that they have been "preserved" with evolution. "Conserved" genes have similar functions in many or all animals. What was yet to be understood, however, was the value of sirtuins.

In 1991, Leonard Guarente, Elysium's co-founder and MIT biologist, along with Nick Austriaco and Brian Kennedy, studied how yeast is aged. Luckily, Austriaco managed to cultivate a variety of yeast strains from samples that he had kept in his fridge for months, generating an atmosphere of tension for the strains. There were only some strains of this sort that could grow here, but Guarente and his team established a pattern: the yeast strains that were best preserved in the refrigerator were also the longest. This guided Guarente so he could concentrate exclusively on these long-lasting yeast strains.

This led to the identification of SIR2 as a gene for yeast longevity. It is important to note that no evidence is available to date that this study can be extrapolated to humans, and further research on the effect of SIR2 on humans is needed. The Guarente's laboratory found that removing SIR2 dramatically reduces the life span of the yeast while increasing the number of copies of the SIR2 gene from one to two significantly increases the life span of the enzyme. But of course, what activated SIR2 still had to be found.

This is where acetyl groups come together. It was initially assumed that SIR2 was a deacetylating enzyme so that acetyl groups could be separated from other molecules, but nobody knew if this was accurate because any attempt to display this function was harmful in a test tube. Guarente and his team were able to figure out that in the presence of nicotinamide adenine dinucleotide, NAD+, in yeast SIR2 could deacetylate other proteins only.

In Guarente's own words: "SIR2 does nothing without NAD+. This was the key finding on the Sirtuin biology arch.

Sirtuins' Future

The research on Sirtuins has been linked mainly to aging and metabolism. "Perhaps 12,000 papers on sirtuins are now available," said Guarente. "The number of papers was in the 100s at the time we discovered NAD+ dependent deacetylase action."

While the sirtuin area continues to grow, fantastic opportunities for research into how triggering sirtuins with NAD+ precursors will lead to more exciting findings can be identified.

RESVERATROL AND SIRTUINS?

Sirtuins are increasing stars in the anti-aging world, and this family of enzymes is illustrated by the University of Wisconsin-Madison.

Why does this matter? Well, if looking graciously younger and older sounds like you're interested, sirtuins are definitely something you ought to recognize.

Sirtuins and their anti-aging functions have been studied since 2001. Many top universities have researched the impact of calorie restriction on prolonged life. The multitude of studies culminated in an interest in a secure link between sirtuins and the length of life.

Recent studies have revealed the enormous potential of anti-aging Sirtuins to further invest heavily in their research growth, with several biotechnology firms. The creation of new drugs for diabetes, Alzheimer's, and other neurological conditions are possible.

Perhaps more exciting is the discovery of groundbreaking anti-aging skincare ingredients through sirtuins for those of us who are worried about wrinkles, fine lines, or some other form of aging.

What is the sirtfood diet and the skinny gene?

Losing seven pounds in 7 days. To be allowed to eat chocolate and to drink coffee and red wine. The Sirtfood Diet appears to be too good to be true, and some warn that it is.

The way you eat activates a group of proteins known as sirtuins or skinny genes. In turn, this is supposed to imitate the effects of exercise and fasting, though Goggins and Matten suggest moderate exercise five days a week for half an hour.

Diet opponents note a lack of proof that the plan will meet its promises. The board-certified diet experts are closed to the idea of slim genes.

Such sirtuin genes have something special about activating the skinny genes. No slim genes exist. You can not enable them. You can't activate them. Some people are metabolically born scrawny and are unable to gain weight.

While they think the diet is overvalued, they are an advocate of encouraging people to eat healthier foods. Here's what you ought to know about the nutrition of Sirtfood.

What is the diet for sirtfood?

The program pushes people to other foods without focusing on items that should be excluded from their diets.

When sirtfoods are consumed, they are processed in the body, removing cell waste and enhancing the functioning of our cells. The product of this burns fat.

If someone eats a diet rich in these types of foods, the result of exercise and fasting is close to that: a leaner, healthy, or healthier one.

What is the dispute?

As far as the science behind sirtuin proteins and this kind of thing are concerned, this is where the trick style enters. The research in humans does not support those claims that it stimulates the "skinny gene" and can improve metabolism and fat intake.

It predicts that the program is not going to fulfill every pledge, but if people consume any of these things, they are going to be better in the long run.

Sirtfood Diet literally sensitizes nature pharmaceuticals; why plant foods are so good for us and how those nutrients are the best that we know are used to improve the functioning of our cells. They are basically the things we can include in our diet as much as possible.

In a London fitness center. We note that 39 of the 40 participants who began Phase 1 of their program (as outlined below) saw an average weight loss of 7 pounds in seven days after muscle gain accounts.

Jampolis has doubts about the trial's legitimacy because they all belonged to the gym: they are a motivated group. He is not the regular Joe Shmoe, who dreams about losing weight on his sofa.

Which are sirts? What are the sirts?

The top 20 dishes are classified as: celery, buckwheat, chilies, coconut, garlic, extra virgin olive oil, green tea, dates Medjool, kale, parsley, red onion, red endive, red wine, soy, turmeric, strawberries, and walnuts.

Jampolis supports the majority of the list, except for the dates for Medjool (it advises that weight restrictions avoid dried fruits) and emphasizes that soya should be minimally processed.

How is the diet organized?

The diet is divided into two levels.

Step 1 lasts a week and restricts calorie intake. On a day of one to three, a maximum of 1000 calories is required per day, and three sirts (flat psol, kale, arugula, celery, fresh ginger, green apple, lemon, and matcha) and one meal should be consumed. For days four to seven, a maximum of 1.500 caloric intake consists of two sirtfood-green juices and two snacks.

The second phase lasts 14 days and comprises three high sirtfoods, a sirtfood green juice and one or two optional sirtfood snacks (including walnuts, dark chocolate or cocoa nibs, Medjool dates, cocoa powder, turmeric, extra virgin olive oil, or a vanilla pod seed or extract and water).

Goggins says Step 1 can be skipped, and people can take "the best course for them."

Jampolis challenges the lack of Phase 2 calorie guidance. She warns, "you may get too much of a good thing," without any limitations.

What else are you going to eat?

Sirtfoods for a meal should be supplemented by protein. The authors recommend oily fish and suggest Strong milk use is perfectly safe..."

"We 're not focusing on what foods are to be cut," explains Goggins. "We do not disseminate food classes," he warns against overloading refined foods, sucrose foods, and mercury-high fish.

Asparagus, green bean, bok choy, blackberries, kumquats, goji berries, raspberries, peanuts, chia seeds, popcorn, cinnamon, ginger, quinoa and are among the foods you have mentioned. They are also supplied in their diet with certain types of meat.

SKINNY THE DIET

Proud as the perfect diet, a Sirtfood diet makes headlines as it encourages red wine and chocolate consumption! Last week, John's mommy (who doesn't have to eat) called him to tell him she bought a book, and she almost breathlessly explained how the diet would help him get skinny genes (He had to put a stop to the urgency of saying that boyfriend jeans are more flattering).

Since the *ethos* is simply about eating for optimal health, he can't help being annoyed if weight loss is all about concentration. In fact, he instinctively considers something "too good to be true." Yet determined to avoid upsetting himself by sweeping testimony from heavy boxers, models, and modern beauty columnists, he soon got stuck with the reading of science.

And what are SIRTs first off?

Sirtuins are a class of proteins found to be involved in fat and glucose metabolism regulation. Evidence also shows that aging, cell death, and inflammation are caused by sirtuins.

SIRT basic research

The work in laboratories has shown that mice at higher SIRT6 levels live longer, and in-vitro trials have shown that SIRT6 can delay human skin cell aging. Certain studies also have shown SIRT2 slows down yeast aging.

What is sirtfood?

The writers highlight the benefits of polyphenol-rich plants. Certain food items include chili, parsley, celery, coffee, wheat, green tea, kale, strawberries, turmeric, red onion, olive oil, and walnuts, as well as red wine and dark chocolate.

Description of Diet

The diet guarantees that you can lose 7lbs in seven days and the loss of weight is fat, not muscle. The caloric intake of the first three days is limited to 1000 Kcal/day consisting of 1 main meal and three green juices (containing parsley, kale, lovage, matcha, celery, and cocktail). For the rest of the week, 2 lunches and two green juices can be eaten every day.

But is it new but fad?

The typical woman who leads a relatively sedentary lifestyle needs about 2000 Kcals; the Sirt diet restricts calorie intake to a half a day, though at the same time promoting daily exercise and gradually reducing calories. Foods on the menu are most nutritious and safe, but only eat one meal a day and live on parsley and kale juice the rest of the day is basically a "crash" diet that carries the possibility of blood sugar destabilization and a slower metabolism. A further risk is that the diet recommends consuming large amounts of raw kale juice – kale is in a group of plants known as brassicas, which can inhibit thyroid function when consumed fresh.

The weight loss is small.

Seven pounds in one week's weight loss is unlikely to reflect long-term body fat shifts. Dietarians eat about 1000 kcal per day for the first three days – about 40%–50 percent of what most people need. Every acute restriction of calorie causes the body, first and foremost, to deplete its stores of glycogen (glycogen is a stored source of carbohydrate in muscle tissue and the liver).

There is a clear relationship between the storage of glycogen and water, while we have deposited about 2 1/2 times the weight of the glycogen in the body! Once our glycogen reserves get exhausted, we lose all the water stored – the quick weight loss. Any inflammation in the body can also contribute to the accumulation of fluid. Most people may not even know that their diet can lead to small but chronic inflammation. Gluten, sugar, alcohol, and even dairy products may cause sensitive individuals to get inflamed. However, a diet that eliminates these foods quickly reduces inflammation and reduces water "on-board!"

Success in Diet

A limited number of committed gym-going dietitians were checked for their diet – not precisely the general population of people pursuing weight loss. How participants were chosen or how variables in behavior and lifestyle were tracked is not clear.

The effectiveness of a diet can not, therefore, be measured meaningfully by observing a specific population group. Moreover, the various variables which can influence outcomes can not be controlled; data collection based on diet remembering and self-reporting leads to high rates of subjectivity and almost guarantees that the results are inexact and data is inaccurate. What is obvious, though, is that calorie limits are an essential part of this diet. Sadly, restrictive diets are often responsible for an increase in appetite-stimulating hormones such as ghrelin. It means that people are left more vulnerable to over-eating and weight gain after food.

Powerful proof

I struggle to see how laboratory experiments with mice, yeasts, and human stem cells provide conclusive evidence that is eating sirtuin-rich foods make you slim, despite re-reading a Chapter titled The Science of sirtuins. While we don't want to harm up to date the exciting and fascinating work on sirtuins, it seems evident that much further research is needed to fully support the theory.

SIRTFOOD AND HACKING OF SIRTFOOD 'THE SKINNY GENE.'

The diet that includes dark chocolate, spinach, red wine, fruits, and coffee? Whether it seems like the perfect way to feel better and lose weight, or it looks too good to be true. Wait, it gets better. These and other so-called "sirtfood" are expected to cause pathways regulated by the "skinny genes" in your body to help burn fat and lose weight, according to the makers of the Sirtfood Diet.

The Sirtfood Diet sounds predictably appealing with a list of tasty items you possibly already love and backed by the news that Adele used it to lose weight after he had a son.

Perhaps you don't want to spoil your chocolate and rot wine here, and maybe science simply does not help the enormous demands of your diet. That is not to suggest that sirtfood is a myth. But, as with all foods that sound too good to be true, with extreme caution, you can look at this one. You need to know here what sirtfoods can and can not do for you.

First and foremost, what's the sirtfood?

Developed by United Kingdom Sirtfood Diet promotes plant-based foods, which are known as "sirtuin activators," for the nutrition pros Aidan Goggins & Glen Matten. Primarily, when you nosh the main ingredients in a diet, you activate proteins encoded with the SIRT1 gene, which Goggins and Matten refer to as "the lean gene."

The role of SIRT1 and sirtuin proteins in aging and longevity is thought to be related to the protective effects of calorie restriction. The argument behind the Sirtfood Diet is that certain foods will activate these pathways through the unlimited sirt diet, "changing fat-burning forces on your body, overloading weight loss and helping to stave off the diseases."

The promotion of Sirtuin-friendly foods alongside dark chocolate, red wine, coffee, fruit, and kale include green matcha tea, extra virgin olive oil, walnuts, red onions, parsley, soja, and turmeric (fantastic aromas and nutritious treats, etc.).

There is some research behind the arguments about the benefits of sirtfoods, but it is very minimal and contentious.

The research at the sirt boundary remains super fresh. Research has explored the function of the SIRT1 gene in aging and survival, the rise in weight associated with aging and aging diseases, and the defense of the heart from high fat dietary inflammation. However, the research is limited to work on test tubes and mice that is not enough to show that sirtuin-improving foods can have weight loss or anti-aging skills in a living, human respiratory body.

The work indicates that the benefits of sirtfood controls may be attributed partly to polyphenol- antioxidant resveratrol, also hypothesized as an item in red wine. "That said, it would not be possible to drink ample red wine to benefit," she said, adding that she also recommends her clients resveratrol supplements.

And some nutrition experts are not keen on how the Sirtfood Diet plan works.

The Sirtfood Diet lacks some essential elements in the safe, balanced diet according to the top dietitians who evaluated the program. Matten and Goggins's diet plan includes three phases: one sirt-food meal and one green juice for some days, take 1 000 calories a day; two sirt-food meals for 1,500 calories for a few days, and two weeks of sirt juices and meals for a total of 1,500 calories.

Keri Gans, RD, author of The Small Change Diet, says she "is not mad at something going on in stages." The shorter periods produce a starvation stage and later on only lead to excessive consumption. "If you limit, at the start of a diet, everyone will lose weight," she says. "But we can't maintain the long-term eating habit."

When you moisturize much without a ton of calories, weight loss is expected, "but typically it's fluid loss," she explains. Therefore, while you can shed pounds on your diet, it's possibly temporary and has no link with sirtuins.

The judgment? Sirtfood is perfect for your health, but not all of it should be.

There is no reason why you can't add sirtfoods to your eating schedule, Alpert says. "I think there is excellent stuff here, such as dark chocolate, red wine, matcha that I love," she said. "I enjoy asking people what to focus on, not what to eat." If it tastes moderate and in a limited quantity is safe, why not?

Gans says she is a fan of many of the foods on the sirt list, including a Mediterranean diet stamp, which is a good standard for scientifically backed balanced eating such as, red wine berries, and olive oil. "I can get rich in polyphenols and antioxidants behind foods," she says.

Blake agrees that the food in the diet is lovely, mainly the trendy ingredients such as turmeric and matcha, which fresh and help make cooking exciting and pleasant to eat. "I see plants that really shine and are packed with phytonutrients," she says. "They are anti-inflammatory, and they are good for you."

All nutrition experts, however, recommend completing the diet with some lean protein and healthy fats, such as nuts and seeds, avocados, and fatty fish such as salmon. In addition to kale and red onions, mix the salad game with more vegetables, spinach, and romaine salad. In the end? Most sirtfood is A-OK and good for you, but don't just swear by the diet to trigger that "skinny gene."

CHAPTER TWO: Sirtfood diet benefits

WHEN EVERYONE SPEAKS ABOUT THE DIET FOR SIRTFOOD

"Sirtfood" looks like something created by aliens, carried to earth intending to acquire mental power and world conquest. Sirtfoods are actually merely foods that are rich in sirtuins. Uh, come again? Come again? Sirtuins are a type of protein that has been shown to control the metabolism of fruit flies and mice, increase muscles and burn fat.

This program will help you lose fat and raise strength, helping your body excel in a long-term loss of weight and a longer, safer, disease-free life. When drinking red wine, all this. Sounds like the perfect diet, right? Okay, before you burn your savings stored in sirtuins, read the advantages and disadvantages.

How does it work?

At its heart, the weight loss is effortless: either increase your calorie burn during your workouts or decrease your caloric intake by creating a calorie deficit. But, what if you could avoid the diet and trigger a "skinny gene" instead without intense calorie restrictions? This is the concept of the Sirtfood Diet by Aidan Goggins as well as Glen Matten, nutrition experts.

Sirtfood is highly nutritious that causes a so-called sirtuin. Matten and Goggins, the "skinny gene" is allowed when energy shortages are produced when calories are limited. In 2003, Sirtuins became interesting in the field of nutrition when researchers noticed that resveratrol, a compound found in red wine, had the same effect on life as calorie restriction, however, it was accomplished without reducing intake. (Find out the absolute truth about the benefits of wine and its health.)

In the pilot study conducted in 2015 (by Goggins and Matten) measuring the efficacy of sirtuins, averaging seven pounds were lost in seven days by 39 participants. The findings are remarkable, but it is important to note that this is a limited sample size observed over a brief period. Experts on weight loss also have concerns about the firm claims. "Studies that concentrate primarily on single species (like yeast) at the cellular level have been highly simplistic and extrapolate statements. The cellular occurrence does not actually correlate to what occurs in the human body at the macro level," said Adrienne Youdim (MD), head of the Center for Weight Loss and Nutrition at Beverly Hills, CA. (Here, find out this year's best and worst diets.)

Which foods are high in sirtuins?

This lists the top 20 high sirtuin foods that seem to be more of a trendy food list than a fresh, sophisticated diet. Examples include red wine, arugula, chilies, green tea, walnuts, dates of Medjool, coffee, turmeric, and the favorite-scale health conscious. While healthier foods are being promoted, weight loss would not automatically be promoted on their own.

What does the diet involve?

The diet is carried out in two phases. Phase 1 lasts three days and limits calories to a thousand per day, including three green juices and a meal that has been approved for sirtfood. Step 2 lasts for four days and raises the average allowance of two green juices and two foods to 1500 calories a day.

During these stages, there is a maintenance program that is not dependent on calories but on small servings, healthy meals, and mainly sirtfoods. The 14-day maintenance schedule involves three meals, one green tea, and one or two sirtfood snacks. Followers are expected to complete 30 minutes of exercise five days a week, but it is not the main objective of the program.

Which are the advantages?

When you follow this diet strictly, you will lose weight. "If you are eating like 1,000 kale calories, 1,000 taco calories, or snickerdoodles of 1,000, your weight will lose by 1,000!" Dr. Youdim says. Yet she also points out that with a more rational calorie limit, you will succeed. The average daily intake of calories from non-diet individuals is 2,000 to 2,200, and reduction to 1,500 is still minimal and, for the most part, a successful weight loss technique.

Are precautions available?

For limited space or substitutions, this method is stringent, and weight loss can only be achieved if the minimum calorie consumption is completed, which makes it impossible to adhere to the long-term requirements. This means that any weight you lose during the first seven days will possibly recover once you stop. Your main concern? "The restriction of protein consumption with juices can lead to the loss of muscle mass. Losing your muscle means lowering your metabolic rate or 'metabolism,' which makes it harder for weight maintenance," she says.

Generally, there are other ways that you can reduce calorie consumption without the food you consume. This says that the diet isn't necessarily "unhealthy," so it won't necessarily warn if a patient succeeds.

If you follow the strategy, make sure you consume plenty of protein and change the foods you consume to avoid deficiencies in vitamins. Our take? The diet is unbelievably strict and has not been sufficiently proven. You are far better off developing a lifestyle that suits your individual needs for a variety of whole foods.

We talk all the time about fad diets here at the specialty food Knowledge Council Site. We usually dismiss them and encourage a healthy eating plan with room for indulgences and celebrations. Often, the diets we speak about are based on some sound recommendations on nutrition, and others we just can not believe exist. We will think about this next diet in the following chapter. The latest on the menu is the sirtfood diet, and we are here to demonstrate to you why you don't need such a limitation in your life. This isn't scientific or sustainable.

The sirtfoods diet is based on the concept of certain foods stimulating sirtuins in your body, different proteins hypothesized for various benefits, from protecting your body's cells from inflammation to aging. The dietary products include blueberries, green tea, dark chocolate, citrus fruits, bananas, garlic, onions, capers, turmeric, and red wine.

Proponents clarify that the diet has two "simple steps". Step one consists of seven days with three sirtfood-packed meal and sirtfood green juices of 1,000 calories per day. You could be marginally less famished on 4 to 7 days when two green juices and two meals will raise your consumption to 1,500 calories. Phew! Phew!

Phase two is less optimistic. This process lasts two weeks, during which, in addition to your particular green juice, you will eat three daily "healthy" sirtfood-rich meals. The aim is to promote further weight loss during this time. While sirtuins' advantages seem promising, the Sirtfood diet is another way to "lose 7 pounds in seven days!" And now you have learned that drastic diets don't work like that.

Weight is a health determinant, but it isn't the only one. Measuring people's health success by losing X pounds in X time ignores all the other advantages of food. Food is full of energy to do things such as exercise, shower, and breathing. This also has nutrients that can facilitate many body functions and is, therefore, a typically enjoyable activity. There is far more to be focused on general health than appearance, and assessing performance in terms of weight loss alone is incomprehensible.

This diet emphasizes a daily intake of 1,000 to 1,500 calories, much less than most people need. If we severely limit our intake of food, our instinctive response is over-drive. Your body is intelligent and treats this lack of support as an assault. We prefer to overcompensate, which is why we can all be "hampered" and thus overspent when we actually have an opportunity to eat. Careful and intuitive cooking is a more reasonable route than food restriction.

While controversial research is being carried out on the benefits of sirtuins, there are few or no research on the particular diet of sirtfood. However, we already have specific recommendations that have been extensively studied and tested for decades. If you forget what "good food" is, it's easier to continue.

It's perfect if you want to include a few sirtfoods in a food program. Foods such as dark chocolate, fruit, green tea, and cups all have their place in a healthy diet! Nonetheless, commitment to a plan with these stringent criteria is impractical and may be detrimental to your food relationship. By implementing a food plan full of variety and careful feeding, you can build healthy, long-term relationships with food. Cheers to that!

How sirtfood diet work?

That was everything you need to learn about the right now, the investment Diet, from research to fresh, tasty recipes to try.

The weight loss of Adele has been talked about by everybody recently, especially after photos of the singer reportedly emerged at the Oscars after the party with seven stones lighter.

This tends to come after photos of the singer on a beach in Anguilla that lost three stones at Christmas.

How did she do it? The Sirtfood diet famous for deliberately allowing those who adopt it to have red wine, and chocolate is obviously taken. In recent years, Sirtfoods diet has been as large as the 5.2 Diet and Dukan diet, popular not only with Adele but with celebrities like Lorraine Pascale or Jodie Kidd. But is it another diet that promises too much, or could it really help you get slim down and feel better following a sirtfood plan?

We spoke to our experts to separate reality from fiction and to show you everything you could want to understand about the Sirtfood Diet.

Sirtuins are the type of protein which protects cells in our bodies from dying or becoming inflamed due to illness, even if the research has shown that they can also help regulate the metabolism, develop your muscle, and also burn fat with this label.

The headlines of the Sirtfood Diet are red wine and dark chocolate because they are both high in sirtuin activators.

Obviously, this is not the entire picture, and the effects will not be felt by lining Merlot and Green and Blacks (more pity).

The Sirtfood Diet plan concentrates on adding healthy sirtfood to your intake.

Ironically, another top dish is coffee, good news if you are fed up with caffeine. Countries where people eat a significant number of sirtfoods also include Japan and Italy, both consistently ranked among the healthiest countries in the world.

Is there a diet schedule for Sirtfood? Yes, there is. No, there is.

1st Week:

- Limit your intake to 1000 calories per day.
- Eat a lavish meal of one sirtfood a day.
- Drink three green juices of sirtfood a day.

2nd Week:

- Up to 1500 calories a day.
- Take two meals full of sirtfood a day.
- Drink two green juices of sirtfood a day.

There is no set path in the long run. This is all about changing your lifestyle to make you feel happier and energized by as many sirtfoods as possible. For more info, see point 5 (below).

Who has the Sirtfood Diet?

The pair of health consultants have always focused on healthy eating and not on weight loss called Aidan Goggins and Glen Matten. The new book "The Sirtfood Diet" features a schedule of three meals a day, supplemented with nutritious sirtfoods, such as buckwheat and stir-fry crumbs or smoked salmon super salads.

Was your diet perfect for Sirtfood?

Rob says one positive thing about your diet is that any food you consume is favorable for you, which means that your total intake of vitamins, minerals, and nutrients is probably high.

He adds, however, that any diet that cuts off whole food groups can be harmful. 'The idea to turn on the 'skinny gene' is not backed by robust studies. The complete Sirtfood diet is very restrictive, both in terms of foods and calories, which can make it challenging to follow too. There is also no evidence that it is more effective than any other calorie regulated diet to lose weight.'

In other words, why not consume foods if you want to lose weight because you are mindful of your total calorie consumption? (And, when you're at our favorite fat-loss breakfast).

Who's not going to try the Sirtfood diet?

Rob says he wouldn't consider following the diet for those with diabetes. Moreover, he adds that it can be difficult if you're extremely involved. If you go ahead, he warns that in the first stage of this plan, he can expect side effects such as headaches or lights as the body adapts to the lower intake.

Recipes for Sirtfood

If you are considering trying the Sirtfood Diet, we're here to give you five delicious recipes from Aidan Goggins and Glen Matten's "The Sirtfood Diet" book, which includes a seven-day plan to lose an average of 7 lb., but adding sirtfood to your diet may also help if you prefer a more calming approach.

The juice of sirtfood

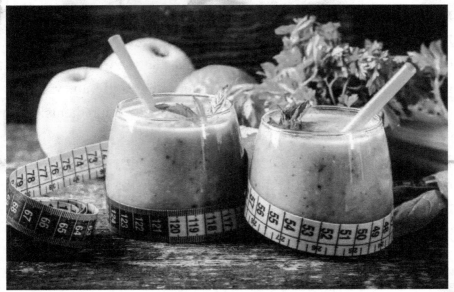

The Sirtfood Juice is an excellent way to start, so we throw the recipe to start as a bonus extra. The book tells you to drink three drinks, add one meal for the first three days, two meals for the next four days, two foods for the next 4.

Foods:

- 2 wide (75 g) kale handfuls.
- ½ standard tsp. green tea matcha.
- Particularly Large multitude of rockets (30 g).
- ½ green medium apple.
- Very small lovage plants (optional) with a handful (5 g).
- A very small flat-leaf parsley (5 g).
- Green celery of 2–3 full twigs (150 g), including its leaves.
- ½ lemon juice.

Directions:

Put together the greens (parsley, kale, lovage, and rocket, if they are being used), and then juice them. We find that the effectiveness of juicers in juicing leafy vegetables can differ significantly, and you can have to re-juicer the rest before moving on to other ingredients. The goal is to get some 50 ml of juice from the greens.

Then add the celery and apple. You can peel the citrus and position it through the juicer as well, but simply squeezing the lemon by hand in the juice is much simpler. You will have a minimum of 250ml of juice at this point, maybe slightly more. Unless the beverage is made and ready to drink, can you add green matcha tea?

Put a few drops of juice into a bowl, then use the matcha or tablespoon to stir vigorously. Matcha is used in the first two drinks of the day only because it contains mild levels of caffeine. This can keep people awake if they are drinking it late (for people not used to this). Remove the rest of the juice until the matcha is dissolved. Give it a final swirl, and you'll drink your juice ready. Feel free to add plain water to your taste.

Muesli sirt (serving 1)

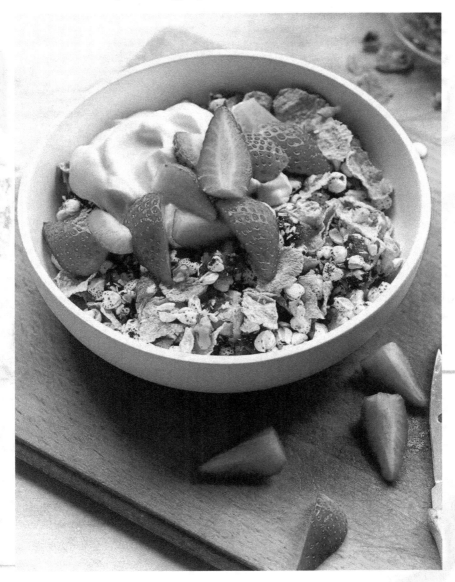

If you want to make this in bulk or prepare it the night before, just mix the dry ingredients and keep it in an airtight jar. All you have to do the next day is to add the yogurt and strawberries, and it's perfect.

Foods:

- 15 g, chopped walnuts.
- 10 g nibs of cocoa.
- 10 g puffs of buckwheat.
- 15 g of cocoa flakes or cocoa desiccated.
- 20 g flowers of buckwheat.
- 100 g of plain Greek yogurt (e.g., soy or coconut yogurt).
- 40 g dates of Medjool sliced and pitted.
- Hulled as well as chopped 100 g of strawberries.

Directions:

Combine the above ingredients (leave the strawberries and yogurt out if they're not immediately served).

Aromatic breast of chicken with kale and red onions, tomato as well as chili salsa (serves 1) Foods:

- 2 tsp turmeric on the ground.
- Chopped 50 g kale.
- 1/4 lemon juice.
- 1 tsp of fresh ginger chopped.
- Extra virgin olive oil 1 tbsp.
- 20 g of sliced red onion.
- 120 g chicken breast without fat.
- Tomato 130 g (approximately 1).
- Buckwheat 50 g.
- Salsa.
- Parsley 5 g thinly sliced.
- 1 chili bird's eye, finely chopped.
- 1 tablespoon capers, excellent cut.

Directions:

To make the salsa, take away the tomato's eye and peel it very well, ensuring as much fluid as possible is maintained. Mix chili, capers, lemon juice, and parsley. You can put it all in a blender, but the outcome is a little different.

Heat the oven to 220°C / gas 7. In 1 teaspoon of turmeric, marinate the lemon juice, the chicken breast, and a little butter. Leave on ovenproof for 5–10 minutes until dry, then add a chicken marinated and cook on either side for a minute or so, until golden yellow, then move to the oven (place on the baking tray when your pan is not ovenproof) for eight to ten minutes or till it cooked. Turn off the heat, cover with foil and leave before serving 5 minutes to rest.

In the meantime, cook the kale 5 minutes in a steamer. With a little olive oil, fry the red onions and ginger, until soft yet uncolored, add the cooked kale and fry another minute. Cook the buckwheat with the remaining teaspoon of turmeric according to the package directions. Serve along with vegetables, chicken, and the salsa.

Bites of Sirtfood (15-20 bites)

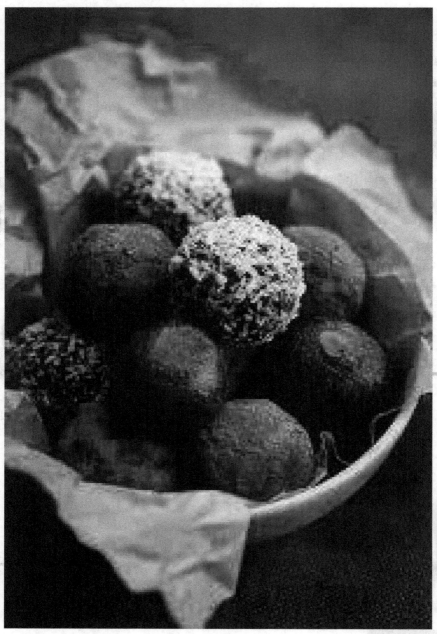

Foods:

- One to two tbsp of water.
- 120 grams of walnuts.
- 250 g dates of Medjool, pitted.
- 30 g dark chocolate (85% solid cocoa), split into pieces;
- 1 tbsp. paste of cocoa.
- Extra virgin olive oil 1 tbsp.
- 1 tbsp. turmeric ground.
- 1 vanilla pod or 1 tsp of vanilla extract scraped.

Directions:

In a food processor, put the walnuts and the chocolate until you have a fine powder.

Remove all the other ingredients except the water and combine until ball forms. Based on the consistency of the mixture, you can or may not apply water – you don't want it to be too messy.

Using your hands to blend into tiny balls and cool in a pan that is airtight for at least 1 hour before feeding. You can roll any of the balls into a little more cocoa or dehydrated cocoa to get a different finish. They can hold in your fridge for up to 1 week.

Asian King stir-fried with noodles of buckwheat (serves 1)

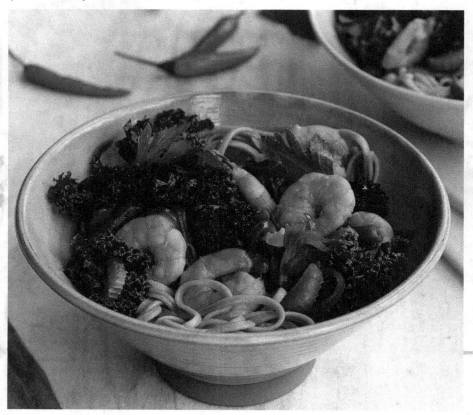

Foods:

- 150 g of raw king prawns shelled, deveined.
- 75 g soba (noodles of sweet wheat).
- 2 tsp. tamari (if you do not avoid gluten, you can use soy sauce).
- 2 tsp. of olive oil extra virgin.
- 1 chili bird's eye, finely chopped.
- 1 clove of garlic, finely chopped.
- 40 g of celery cut and sliced.

- 1 tsp. of fresh chopped ginger.
- 20 g of sliced red onions.
- 50 g spinach, chopped roughly.
- 5 g celery or lovage leaves.
- 75 g of chopped green beans.
- Chicken stock 100ml.

Directions:

Steam a frying pot over high heat, then cook the prawns for 2-3 minutes in one teaspoon tamari and one teaspoon oil. Move the prawns to a plate. Wipe out the pan with kitchen paper, because you can need it again.

Cook the noodles 5-8 minutes in boiling water or as instructed. Drain and reserve.

In the meantime, cook the garlic, chili and red onion, ginger, beans, celery, and kale in the remaining oil for 2–3 minutes over medium-high heat. Add the stock and boil, then cook until the vegetables are tender, but still crunchy, for about a minute or two.

Put the prawns, noodles, and celery or lovage leaves in the pan, carry back to the boil, then take off the heat and serve.

Strawberry Stool Buckwheat

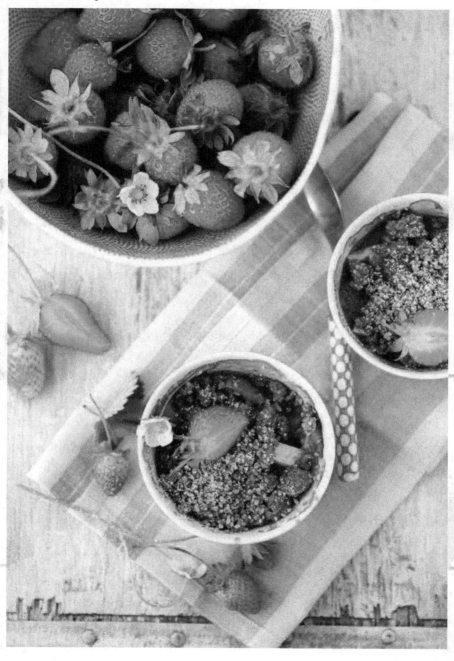

Foods:

- 1 tbsp. turmeric ground.
- 80 g avocado.
- ½ lemon juice.
- Tomato 65 g
- 25 g Dates of Medjool, pitted.
- Buckwheat 50 g.
- Extra virgin olive oil 1 tbsp.
- 1 caper tbsp.
- Parsley 30 g.
- 20 g onion red.
- Hulled 100 g strawberries.
- Rocket 30 g.

Directions:

Cook buckwheat in turmeric as directed by the packet. Drain and hold cold on one foot.

Chop the dates, tomato, avocado, red onion, capers, and parsley thoroughly, and mix in the fresh buckwheat. Slice the strawberries and add oil and lemon juice to the salad gently. Serve on a rocket bed.

If you want to give the Sirtfood diet but have little time (or cooking skills), the company behind the diet has launched a delivery service that provides you with the option to follow the scheme, minus all cuts.

How does the sirtfood diet help you to burn fat?

While the world is waiting for Adele to drop new music, her weight is only a little obsessed. It looks fantastic (well, didn't it always?) and it's said to be the Sirtfood Diet.

The 19-year-old at Hingham, Massachusetts, Lexi Larson said she had met Adele on holiday in Anguilla and also that the celebrity musician said she had "lost about a hundred pounds," which she characterized as "a very positive experience."

So what is the Sirtfood Diet big deal?

The diet is based on polyphenols, which are natural compounds in plant foods that help protect cells in the body from infection or death by disease. It depends on a specific list of healthy, polyphenolic foods, the Sirtfood Diet promises a reduction in weight and fat without the loss of muscle.

What is the plan? What is the program?

The Sirtfood diet has two phases; the first lasts one week, and the second lasts two weeks. During the early three days of the program, the sum of one meal of sirtfood and three green juices is limited to 1,000 calories. Two green sauces and two sirtfoods can be eaten daily for the remainder of the first week. During Phase Two, three sirtfood meals and one green juice are part of the daily meal plan.

Following three weeks of 'jumpstart,' Goggins and Matten suggest keeping sirtfood in their meals to keep getting progress.

What promises it?

During the first week, (without losing muscle mass) if you don't deviate from the plan, the Sirtfood Diet promises a weight loss of seven pounds. To help boost the memory and regulation of blood sugar and reduce the risk of chronic diseases, it also appears to have anti-aging effects."

But does it bring about?

Sirtuin's function work is fragile, mainly laboratory studies involving yeast, laboratory animals, and human stem cells. One research suggests the same beneficial impact on human metabolism as that of calorie restriction on polyphenol intake. Yet it is difficult to tell with absolute certainty whether people will do so, until such time, this dietary strategy is successfully evaluated in human clinical trials.

What can you eat?

While individual meals are frequent in any supermarket or health food shop (and may even be in your kitchen), it may not be easy for others to find.

Sirtfood is spinach, red wine, dark chocolate, cocoa powder, currants, capers, onions, garlic, walnuts, and strawberries. Most of the ingredients can be found quickly and are known as healthy choices. However, additional components such as buckwheat, lovage, and matcha green tea could be harder for the source.

What can you not eat? What can you not eat?

Officially, the Sirtfood Diet does not ban food, but it is especially severe during the initial three days when you are limited to 1,000 calories.

Are there any disadvantages?

The most challenging aspect of the Sirtfood diet is calorie restriction and reliance on green juice, which can be unhealthy for some groups of people. For people with medications like coumadin, or with health problems like diabetes, she does not prescribe this diet. You will also miss it if you're running or pregnant or breastfeeding extensively.

In general, I do not advocate diets based on overly restrictive external guidelines. Many of the suggested sirtfoods, however, are health-promoting, and I would recommend that people include them in their meals.

SIRTFOOD DIET IS NOW A WEIGHT LOSS SCHEME THAT HELPS YOU TO DRINK RED WINE AND DARK CHOCOLATE.

We claim to be fast to lose weight, promising to help people to lose like seven pounds in 7 days. Another distinctive feature of the diet is that it contains more indulgent foods, such as dark chocolate and red wine, along with conventional, healthy alternatives, such as kale, strawberries, and all other food.

While the diet claims to put its participants in a fast way to lose weight, it also encourages extreme calorie restriction. Here's what you need to learn before you pursue the Sirtfood Diet.

The Sirtfood Diet consists of natural compounds found in so-called polyphenols in fruit and vegetables. Goggins and Matten say that certain polyphenols mimic the effects of fasting and exercise by stimulating proteins called sirtuins in our bodies.

Also referred to as SIRTs or silent information regulator sirtuins play a role, particularly during periods of fasting or extreme heat restrictions, in how the body metabolizes sugar and stores fat.

Research published in the International Journal of Molecular Sciences in 2016 showed that obesity could be controlled. Nevertheless, the evidence is in the early stages, and most research comes not from human studies but animals or human cells.

The Sirtfood Diet suggests that Goggins and Matten consume a lot of foods rich in polyphenols to cause sirtuins in the body. Such foods are called 'sirtfoods' hence the name of the diet. Nonetheless, researchers are still studying exactly how polyphenols affect sirtuins in the body and whether they can potentially support weight loss.

I could find no experimental evidence that the Sirtfood Diet works by stimulating sirtuin proteins.

The foods suggested will certainly stimulate sirtuins, but that doesn't mean that it is purely because of that that you lose weight. You lose weight primarily due to calorie restrictions initially and 'reasonably' balanced eating.

All in the plan is listed in the Sirtfood Diet book.

Adherents to the diet plan may also expect to drink several sirtfood full juices that include ingredients such as arugula, kale, ginger, pot parsley, green apple, and matcha powder. The juice is all vegetables and fruits. Drink it, there is no harm.

But definitely, it is not the best idea to change that with a meal. Drinking only food juice will cause a blood sugar spike, as the juice has little to no fiber insoluble. Occasionally the blood sugar spike does not hurt, but over time, it may lead to health problems such as insulin resistance and prediabetes if you have chronically elevated blood sugar levels.

In the sense of replacement, on the other hand, it will be very safe. Rather than consuming a sweetened beverage and added sugar, such as soda, it is a safer option to choose the water.

The diet's founders say that the tens of thousands of people who have tried the diet have found rapid and sustained weight loss successful. Nevertheless, Baylin says that any caloric diet is always successful in the short term.

"In the short term, you'll probably lose weight if you eat fewer calories," she says. And though she admits that you can lose fat by mixing your diet with exercise, you're "most likely" to lose water weight after going on your diet.

The Academy of Nutrition and Dietetics recommends between 1,600 and 2,400 calories a day for women and between 2,000 and 3,000 calories for men a day. And you'll lose weight on any diet that requires only 1000 calories a day but doesn't mean that it's safe or healthy.

In addition to being nutritionally healthy or calorie-adequate, Baylin says the diet is safe. "Nothing in the foods suggested is harmful, all of which are absolutely safe.

But in the first phase of strict caloric restraint, I would not recommend it. However, most healthy adults should have no problems following this diet.

The problem is that a diet is simply a diet, so if people do not eat healthily in a way that is a new way of life, but a "punishing" diet, they will never get to eat healthily so marginally less and regain the weight.

The jury also does not know if the diet has a long-term impact, and if it may have problems with other health conditions.

Diagnostics, however, warn that people with diabetes or other medical disorders may have significant health risks in this diet. Therefore, it is always recommended to ask a doctor about the possible risks before undertaking a highly restrictive diet, such as the Sirtfood Diet.

How to build a diet plan that works?

Below are two free diet plans. They're very basic, but don't make a mistake, and they're proven to lose weight effectively. You don't even have to make this diet exactly as describe it. Use them as a guide and create a better plan. Read this now, so you cannot stop STARTING TODAY this weight loss battle.

Free Working Diet Plans

The diet for a protein shake

It might not be appropriate for everybody. But if you really want to lose weight quickly AND safely, this works very well. If you are strict on this, you will literally lose 20 pounds a month. All you have to do is to drink protein shakes all day long. Girls drink 4 of them, usually Men, 5. Women, 5. One important thing to remember is to apply fiber to them to hold you full.

Two things to keep this kind of diet in mind. If you don't put something like a banana or apple into the protein shakes, your carbs will be reduced. So I would eat 1-2 apples in this program as snacks. You 're still short in dietary fats. I suggest you add 1 Virgin Olive Oil tablespoon to 2 of your protein shakes so that this program will contain some good fats.

The diet includes eggs and black beans

This diet basically revolves around eggs or 1/2 can of black beans at your dinner. So if you eat three meals, you have to be one of those things at each meal. You can choose, so you don't feel suffocated. Black beans are high in protein and fiber, while the content of the eggs is small. Both options fill you up, are cheap and healthy.

Here are two free diet plans. Using or change them if the weight loss is pleasant and straightforward.

Why Are Diets Not Working?

When you're one of the almost 160 million overweight Americans, you're probably looking for a single diet plan to help lose some extra pounds. Day by day, customer by customer, Jane hears of the desire to lose weight, and almost everyone tells her about their diets.

Sadly, almost everyone asks her first how the diet succeeded, and then the importance returned. Did this happen to you? If you say honestly to have success with a diet at first, you're not alone to gain weight again. Nearly every person who has tried to "die" gets load back. If you are overweight, you probably have another health condition as well. High cholesterol, elevated triglycerides, high blood sugar, cancer, heart disease, coronary artery disease, and other obesity-related health issues.

It has helped people lose weight and overcome chronic health issues, a magic bullet to master weight loss, and associated health conditions also need to be identified. You'll hear about the new drug that can help you lose weight, and you might even have tried it yourself. Yet there is a side effect ALWAYS. EVERYTHING. All medications have side effects. You should remove medicines from the weight loss program.

Currently, there is far more than just hope. The best way of weight loss is by adopting a balanced lifestyle. In fact, the safest way to lose weight and cope with chronic health conditions is by dietary changes from all leading health organizations such as the Centers for Disease Control, the World Health Organization, the American Heart Association, the American Cancer Association, and many others.

How are adaptations to the lifestyle? Simply put, changes in lifestyles are a "way of life." Do these three things if you want a healthy life. (i) A healthy diet (ii) Exercise 30 minutes a day (iii) Have the right mentality. Bring these three basic things into your daily routine, and you'll change your life.

Let's give you quick ideas for each of the three things that you should do every day to lose weight and become healthy.

Eat a balanced diet-Add in your diet more fruit and vegetables. Fruits and vegetables contain fiber, and fiber is essential for good intestinal health, which is crucial for good overall health.

When you can, eat one salad a day. Fill it with cucumbers, lettuce, celery, olives, tomatoes, broccoli, carrots, or your favorite foods. Salads are not just a fantastic way to get your vegetable parts, and they are full of nutrients. Foods that contain high water also help combat fat. When most people screw up, too much clothing is applied. Remember that a dressing tablespoon may have more than 150 calories. Go to the dressing quickly to save calories.

If you want to eat meat, you can eat chicken (free-range organic, as available), fish (particularly deep-fished, wild fish like snapper, halibut, salmon, and turkey). If you want to try, alternative meats look into buffalos, ostriches, and other sports.

Improve your intake of whole grains. Wholesale grains can be found in so many food items that your daily consumption can be easily increased.

Drink plenty of good clean water, because most people don't know about this natural but essential item from any good weight loss program. Water's necessary for so many biological processes in the human body, yet not enough; you actually undermine your health. You don't have to waste any wealth on a special filter, either.

Get a bit of exercise every day, notice a little practice. You don't have to train for the Iron Man to be healthy. Depending on your conditioning level, simply walking for 30 minutes daily will change your health. One of the reasons many people don't start a training program is because they think they have a big commitment, and it's an excuse.

Have the right mental attitude, which is particularly important during this period of challenging economics. Note that you begin with your mood and your way of seeing life. If you are self- defeated, you will find yourself in several other facets of your life. If you have difficulty thinking about yourself, your life, and your future, you can still go to it.

A safe life and happier life can be yours with a few easy lifestyle changes. Note, the steps to a healthier lifestyle are eating a decent diet.

DIET PLAN WHICH DROPS WEIGHT

Who's ever out or knows someone who's adopted a new diet? After perhaps losing 10 to 20 pounds, you get sidetracked, and the diet goes by and by. This is the most interesting part. You get the pounds you lost within a short space of time and add an additional five or ten as a door prize.

First, because you can't keep weight off and second, you can do something that works. The trick to believing what the reader has to say is to understand and accept that nothing can be achieved by telling you this.

Let us start by examining the many diets that are plastered throughout the internet and magazines. For the apparent reason, we won't mention names, but who they are is simply an issue in your kitchen cupboards.

First, we must look at what these purchased diets do. We would be the first to say that in these different plans, people are actually losing weight. It's a big one sometimes, but what do we do to our bodies? Will these diets teach us to keep our portions under control? Do they shrink our stomachs naturally? No to both questions.

The biggest thing we need to look at is, how much money does this diet make, and who does it? In today's world, a pretty safe bet seems that when something sounds good on the surface comes along, someone makes money from it.

So, many doctors did you see because of your weight, that told you how to shed the pounds successfully? How many nutritionists have you visited who have shown you how to lose weight successfully and the program? How long would they be in business if they said nothing more than what you are paying for food now?

Something like this is the DIET CONSPIRACY. Press such as magazines, the internet, and newspapers advertise people who do not lose weight. They are nothing more than guilt travel agents. The category will include Hollywood.

The food industry makes food that adds centimeters to the waistline. Where a secret ingredient is used in potato chips, which stimulates our desire to eat the next, and the following before the bag goes out. Restaurants contain sections well beyond the needs of our bodies. Groceries have delights that make your taste buds mad as you push through the window. Of course, you'll be tempted to buy something that smells so good.

Doctors beat their patients over the weight, but how many of them teach us how to hold the pounds off? How much money is generated from stomach stapling procedures, when you mention doctors? How many physical issues are caused by food?

How large is the food industry? All medications, powders, packaged meals, snacks, cookbooks, weekly meetings are included, the list goes on and on. Millions of dollars, maybe trillions, are invested by the country. Tell yourself, is it really beneficial for these businesses to lose weight once and for all and keep it away? And is it free, whatever they promote?

We definitely do not want to exclude many fitness centers and sports equipment providers. We almost hesitate to include them, because many people use these to tone their bodies and hold their weight off. You must admit that exercise is often a way of throwing out the pounds.

Now, looking at all this stuff, do we really assume that the many people mentioned here really seem to our advantage? If that was the case, why can't people lose weight and keep it away? How do so many people in their wardrobe have different types of clothing? Should it be that they know that their weight is going to increase soon?

The conspiracy theory is that all weight loss plans are aimed at people who do not hold weight away. The growth of the companies listed is making a small contribution to keeping the public overweight. How else would they worship the Almighty Dollar at the feet of their God? You will keep the customer coming if you want to get another taste of the fruit.

Please, I don't want to say doctors don't know how to help us lose the pounds. So often was it meant when it was parting, "You have to lose weight." When you heard it said, "You have to lose weight, and here is exactly how to do so?"

This food plan requires you to treat every meal with a certain degree of preparation and anticipation. Mostly the food schedule is either i) you no longer consume eight ounces of food per meal and ii) you consume three hours apart. It's no okay cheating or eating high-fat things and expects to lose weight. Two powers are at stake here. The first is the ounces of food and time, and the second is how the body responds to it.

Let's try and offer an instance. A car uses the same fuel as our blood. You go to the gas station and buy the same fuel as you eat. The fuel purchased is used to drive a certain distance. The food we consume is used to fuel our bodies for any mission.

Below are the ends of the parallels. The leftover fuel is stored in the gas tank when the car journey is made. When the body is finished for the day, the remaining fuel is still saved, so it is fat for future use that day instead of stored in a tank. The following day more fuel is added, and the fat is stored. That should be quite easy to understand.

Common sense must be practiced if this eating program is implemented. Many parents do it for their fun. Dad's already lost about 40 pounds. Everybody knows that women lose weight a little harder than men, but Mom is very pleased with their own growth. There will always be a community of people who can't recognize everything that says about faith. We say that we know correctly what works and why. It is definitely not a negative thing, especially given today's floating misinformation. Small foods also improve metabolism and regulate blood sugar.

The lower you hold your blood sugar, the lower your insulin would be. A fact that insulin is the fat-bonding element. If you keep your blood sugar steady, your level of insulin should be natural so that fat is not stored in excess around your heart.

Every meal is just eight ounces, but healthy eating can be accomplished after a while. In reality, 8 ounces every 3 hours will fill you after a short time. It's a must to drink plenty of water or similar beverages. No sugar drinks, no soda pop, and no sucrose drinks are recommended.

It is essentially three 8-ounce servings of chocolate milk consumed at crucial points all day long: A second after you wake up and a third after your workout. That's what it is and why it's so simple. Yet is this the free ticket to eat as much chicken as you want all day long? Sadly, not, but combined with a balanced diet, it will help you to quickly lose a lot of belly fat.

The explanation of why milk is such a good is then clarified. Fat-free milk doesn't count against you and helps if you are hungry between food. It's hard to label them foods if you consume five or six times a day.

The body requires vitamin D for the use of calcium out of milk. To use the calcium out of milk, the organization has to use a bit of fat to use vitamin D. The 1 percent fat is only enough to do that. Until now, for some dad, at least 1 percent did not cause difficulties at the scale.

A big glass of 1% chocolate, one tablespoon of "Dutch Chocolate" powder (acquired in bulk in most grocery stores selling volume) and around pine Stevia Teaspoon, a natural replacement for sugar. Sugar doesn't bode well in the weight loss scheme, so why use it?

Just put a little milk in the glass and combine the chocolate and stevia and then add the rest of the liquid. When you have to blend the mixture, then it will be easier to have a larger jar. Use smaller bottles for this process. It is much cheaper than purchasing shop-bought chocolate milk, and a lot safer.

ENJOY YOUR DINING WITHOUT RUINING THE DIET PLAN

Yes, the great mystery of food. You are making great strides in achieving your goals for weight loss. You follow your diet plan by letter, you regularly practice, and you have seen a relatively rapid loss of weight. But you're invited to eat with friends or family every now and then, or you just love some good Italian food. Then what about the days you're out and about and just don't have time for a home-cooked meal?

Many people believe that dinner leaves only one option: avoid the diet. Yet here, let's be realistic. You will have some severe damage to your waistline if you dine out two to three times a week (relatively healthy for most people)-and drop out of diet every time.

But here is the good news: diet and exercise can go hand in hand. It can take a little preparation and a great deal of determination, but you can make it work if you are serious about weight loss. Let's think about strategy, then.

Plan the meal before you leave

While this is not always possible, most restaurants nowadays have an online menu. Look at the different options available and choose the diet-friendly ones. If you get ready to order at the restaurant, you're not as tempted by what others order.

Have some protein before you head out

If you get to the ravenous restaurant, all your control will probably fly out of the window. You will finally overeat all the wrong stuff. When you head out, take your bottom off your hunger, consume a little protein-packed snack like a handful of almonds, a boiled egg, or a slice of fatty cheese.

Avoid extras Avoid

Many places placed an extra bread or chips basket on the table before the meal. All these processed carbs and deep-fried chips pose a danger to any diet, so do anything possible to avoid them. When you are with your family or close friends, see if you can prevent the basket completely. When you can't entirely eliminate the temptation, at least sit as far as you can so that you don't nibble before the meal.

Thunder the hunger

Thirst is also confused by hunger, so a large glass of water before your food arrives. Whether or not your body needs food, with all the water in your belly, you can feel less hungry.

Be careful a sugar drink can harm as much as an unhealthy food option. Therefore, alcohol stimulates your appetite and makes you feel thirsty. Keep out of sodas, spirit, and sometimes lemonade. Only stick to water and eat a little lemon. If you want a beer or a cocktail, have one after the meal is over.

Swap your dressing for a soup or salad

The majority of menu appetizers are deep-fried and filled with fat, calories, and sodium. Anything crispy or fluffy is a bad idea, so skip the choices. Take a soup or salad instead.

Soups and salads are high foods for your diet. They will fill you while you are waiting for your entrance, so your body is already quite satisfied by the time it arrives. If your hunger is saturated, you are less likely to overdo it.

Also note, avoid thick soups or dressings when ordering a soup or salad. All that is fluffy would be filled with fats in order for a creamy vegetable soup or just a broth or a drink for your soup. If appropriate, use an olive oil vinaigrette for your dressing.

Get sauces on your side

Restaurants usually have heavy hands with sauces and clothing, so that could be a nightmare for your diet program. If you ask for your sauces and dressings on your side, you can tell how much you are consuming and monitor your diet.

You can also take a smart tip from Tyra Banks: Just dip your bucket's tip-in sauce and dress before every piece. You get all the delicious goodness of a dress without all the sugar and cholesterol.

Caution against sly fats

You may have wisely selected an entrance to fish or chicken. While these are decent choices for low fat, beware of sly fats. Fish is excellent, but if it is not fried fish or tartar slathered fish. Chicken is small in fat but not pounded, fried, or smothered with gravel or cheese. Ask your server how to cook meat and leave fatty sauces or dressings away or, if appropriate, choose something else.

Mind the risks and falls of pasta

Who doesn't like a big Fettuccini Alfredo bowl or a creamy, carbohydrate dish? All the noodles are filled with a walloping calorie count, not to mention the creamy, buttery sauce.

When you have to indulge, pick a tomato or pesto based sauce like we do all from time to time. You will minimize calories and fat considerably while still fulfilling your appetite.

Tell your server for food and substitutes.

When you are uncertain of the dietary efficiency of an item on your menu, don't be afraid to ask your server. You might also know how an element is prepared or any sauces or sides that can be added or omitted. Also, if the server is inexperienced, they're usually happy to consult with the chef (of course, if you inquire nicely).

Many restaurants require fair food substitutions. Ask if you should have a vegetable or baked potato instead of having fried with your grilled chicken breast.

Employ the component sizes

Finally, remember that moderation is an essential factor in an adequate diet. Excessive food choices are still a poor choice. A helpful method to avoid extra food is to get your to-go box before the meal. Place the food you want to eat right away and save the rest for later. You are likely to eat much or all of it if the entire meal is on the plate, but if any of it is put away, it is more likely that you stick to a nutritional section.

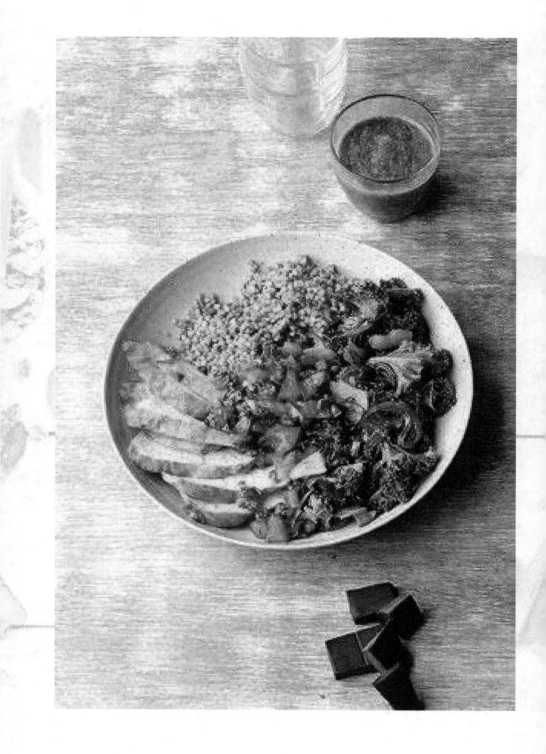

CHAPTER THREE: Sirtfood list

TOP SIRTFOODS

- Capers.
- Buckwheat.
- Celery.
- Kale.
- Extra Virgin Olive Oil.
- Chocolate.
- Chili.
- Lovage.
- Red Wine.
- Coffee.
- Red Onion.
- Red Chicory.
- Strawberries.
- Green Tea – ideal matcha.
- Soy.
- Walnuts.
- Rocket.
- Medjool Dates.
- Turmeric.
- Parsley.

Just a reminder of the science behind the Sirtfood diet program.

Sirtfood is an innovative way to optimally activate our sirtuin genes.

Those are the beautiful foods rich in unique natural plant chemical substances, known as polyphenols, which can activate and unlock our Sirtuin genes. These basically mimic the effects of fasting and exercise and offer remarkable advantages by helping the body to regulate blood sugar levels, burning fat, building muscle, and improving health and memory.

Since they are stationary, plants have established a powerful, sophisticated stress reaction mechanism and manufacture polyphenols to help them respond to environmental challenges. We also absorb these polyphenol nutrients when we eat these plants. This has a profound effect: this stimulates our own intrinsic receptors for stress response.

Although all plants have stress response systems, only some have evolved to produce exceptional amounts of sirtuin-activating polyphenols. Such plants are foodstuffs. Their discovery means that there is a groundbreaking new way to trigger the sirtuin genes, instead of a strict fasting regimen or challenging training programs: eating a diet rich in Sirtfoods. The best thing about your diet is putting (sirt) food on your plate and not removing it.

After the diet and maintenance

We are living in a community where it's desirable to be thin. We idolize individuals who are the most delicate of 5 to 10 % of the population. We are also a country with "super-sized" pieces, interestingly.

Maintenance and Weight loss are the foundations of good living and good health. Stroke, Type II diabetes, cancer, heart disease, depressed mood, obstructive sleep apnea, and more are associated with obesity. For the most part, life facts should be weight management and weight loss.
But many people do not necessarily want to lose weight or sustain weight loss. Weight loss and weight maintenance are hard work, and practical approaches rely on how much a person wants to lose weight.

Some people can effectively exercise and eat alone, and others need invasive interventions such as surgery. And even for those who are fortunate enough to achieve their desired weight, maintenance can be much harder than the initial weight loss, albeit more straightforward.

Loss of weight: Diet and exercise

The weight status of a person is best measured by the Body Mass Index (BMI). Body Mass Index is a calculation that divides the weight of a person by kilograms into square meters. A Body Mass Index calculator is available on the online of national health institutes for the calculation- averse.

According to the Health and Human Services Department, people with Body Mass Index's between 18.5 and 24.9 are considered average weight. People with BMIs from 25 to 29.9 are deemed overweight. People with BMIs from 30 to 39.9 are listed as obese. Eventually, individuals with BMIs over 40 are listed as morbidly obese.

Self-control strategies are an excellent place to begin for Americans who are actually overweight. Medical care is usually reserved for obese or overweight people who suffer from medical conditions or who also have self-managed dieting. Although exercise is necessary for any weight loss or weight maintenance regime, research has shown that dieting is the most efficient method of losing weight. A healthy diet is a balanced and calorie-restricted diet.

What does "limited calories" mean? The Basal Metabolic Rate (BMR) is distinctive to all. BMR is known as the minimum number of calories needed to maintain a comfortable life. This depends on the age, level of biology, operation, and sex (men have BMR higher than women). For example, a bodybuilder from Mr. Universe has a BMR that can calculate that of a senior citizen in a bed. To lose weight, a person must consume fewer calories than their BMR or maintain a diet equal to their lowest caloric requirements and burn down enough calories to undermine their BMR.

According to the USDA, the balanced, caloric diet best approximated to the average American BMR consists of six to seven-ounce of bread, rice, cereal, and grain; three cups of milk, two cups of fruit, and about six ounces of seafood, meat, poultry, nuts, and beans. The USDA has developed resources that help people to determine a diet best matched by their own BMR by height and weight.

All diets must be balanced because not all food types are identical in terms of comparable calories. For example, a high-calorie diet in trans-fats can benefit the heart and help to turn the dietary fat into body fat. A healthy diet is a high fiber diet that is low in saturated or animal fat (fresh fruit and vegetables). Trans fats, which are commonly present in fast and junk food should be absolutely avoided.

So what about the Atkins or South Beach diets? Fad diets such as Atkins and South Beach usually serve as fast-fixed panaceas. Few dieters can maintain the loss of weight from such a dramatic dietary change. Most people just consume meat and vegetables so long before they stick to sweets and cakes. Health researchers found that people would restrict their eating habits only for a short period until they want a healthier diet.

Exercise is also relevant for overweight people who want to lose weight. Training is "yin" to the "yang" diet. The practice raises people's MRB, improves morale, maintains healthy muscles, calories burn out, and avoids diseases such as diabetes and high cholesterol. The health and physical needs of the person preparing to work out should be taken into account in every exercise program. A reasonable place to start is to walk 150 to 200 minutes a week (30 minutes a day).

There's an individual weight loss psychology. Using our perception of our world can make our desire to lose weight easier. Health professionals and specialists on weight loss have dedicated their careers to learning what works and what doesn't. Just a few hints from a long list of useful "mind tricks":

- ✓ Logs and contracts: Those people who are willing to lose weight should keep notes of how much they eat and how much they exercise. Logs help bring it all into perspective and help dietitians prepare what they need to do. Diet and fitness plans also enable people to lose weight. By writing a contract in a concise and specific language, people are obliged to devote themselves or others (e.g., another equal- minded dieter) to weight loss.

- ✓ Stimulus Control: Certain conditions are used as keys or stimuli for unconscious feeding. Great examples of mindless eating behaviors are watching "American Idol" in front of the TV or playing video games. Dieters can restrict their food to one area of the building, such as a kitchen or a dining room.

- ✓ Changing the feeding act: Most people eat too quickly. When people eat fast, they don't know that they're already full. Dietitians must slow down and enjoy their food.

- ✓ Social support: The island is no dieter. This is best to get assistance from friends and family when they lose weight.

✓ Yet, most diets eventually fail. Individuals often underestimate their calorie consumption and seek to meet unattainable weight loss targets. Worst of all, dietitians often gain weight over and above what they lost. Many individuals have a long history of poor diets and persistent weight loss and weight gains. Many struggling dieters benefit from more rigorous nutritional strategies and weight loss, such as weight watchers or healthcare professional supervision. Some can have to take more invasive steps.

Loss of weight: Drugs and "go under the knife."

Many people can not get the desired health and beauty results out of diet and workout alone. There are other possibilities.

Some obese people between 30 and 40 years of age with BMI are eligible for drug therapy. "Pills" contain antidepressants, stimulants, and drugs such as Orlistat that minimize dietary fat absorption. At most, medications contribute only to mild weight drops of 10 % to 15% and end when a patient starts taking medicines. For a fact, both drugs have side effects and no individual weight loss tablets. For example, stimulants are only recommended for short-term use because of their high addiction potential.

Bariatric surgery is the safest treatment for people with moderate obesity or obesity over BMI 35 who have medical conditions such as sleep apnea, diabetes, or coronary-artery disease. The bariatric procedure has shown a dramatic change in the quality of life and curbed medical problems such as cardiac failure, diabetes, and sleep apnea. Bariatric surgery has two types: malabsorbent and restrictive.

Specific bariatric procedures, including the laparoscopic gastric band (LAP-BAND), are the most common option for most patients with morbid obesity. Restrictive bariatric procedures raising the stomach volume and help people feel quicker. The LAP-BAND operation requires the positioning of an elastic band by a highly trained surgeon around the top of the stomach. Procedures such as LAP-BAND have no medical effects and less than 1% of all people who undergo these procedures later die. The qualification for the LAP-BAND is not easy and depends on insurance companies, but most carriers require a history of failed dietary and exercise efforts and batteries of health visits with psychiatrists, nutritionists, and other health professionals.

Anyone who wants to experience the LAP-BAND should also be prepared for a long commitment. After the operation, the band must be rigorously preserved. However, LAP-BAND is an excellent option for those who want to gradually lose a large amount of weight and maintain this weight loss.

Malabsorption bariatric operations such as "Roux-en-Y" are more successful, leading to more loss of weight but riskier. Patients undergoing surgery have their intestines separated by a surgeon to mess with food absorption. Upon surgery, patients must be vigilant to take adequate nutrient replacements and consume other forms of food.

In contrast to LAP-BAND, the malabsorption bariatric procedure is permanent and has a higher risk of medical complications caused by a bowel obstruction, food deficiency, and infection.

Weight maintenance: The hardest way Therefore, you've lost weight or are content with the weight, you just have to keep it. But weight maintenance is difficult in this land of plenty. Candy bars tend to grow out of convenience stores and McDonald's line along every big road. What is John Q. Public health-conscious to do?

Maintaining a safe, balanced diet and exercise schedule is now more critical than ever. Lifelong vigilance is essential. Cosmetic treatments, such as liposuction, may also lead to the elimination and contour of subcutaneous fat.

As with weight loss, there is a weight management psychology:

✓ Visual indications: Health researchers, especially "Mindless Eating: How We Eat More" author, Dr. Brian Wansink, found that people do not eat their stomachs with their eyes. For example, Dr. Wansink discovered that people with a "bottomless" soup bowl eventually consumed 73% more soup than they could otherwise have. Furthermore, they didn't feel sated any more after doing so. Absent a reference point like an empty dish, people just eat. Anyone who wants to maintain their weight should take advantage of this simple psychological strategy by buying little plates, smaller cups, 100-calorie "snack" packets, and totally avoiding buffets all- you-can-eat.

- ✓ Taking a day off: Health researchers have found that if people are physically healthy, they are more likely to feed. Researchers feed obese subjects and physically suit a milkshake in a quaint experiment, and then gave them as much ice cream as they needed. The smaller subjects who are usually limited to food warned of the wind and consumed more ice cream than their obese counterparts. This line was inspired by the popular suggestion that everyone would undergo strict dietary maintenance one day a week. Rather than eating a chocolate bar every other day, people trying to avoid weight would enjoy a bowl of ice cream and a few cookies every Sunday night after the Simpsons.

All manages their own fate in terms of weight loss and maintenance. We all must remember that healthy living is regulated by us. Determination is essential for proper loss and maintenance of weight. We all hold the keys to our own safer, slimmer selves.

Shopping list for Sirtfood diet

This seems like a crazy question, but have you ever wondered how you eat? Sure, you might say, of course. You go to the shop, have a cart, put in food, pay, and take it home. All right, but do you ever notice that you spend more time than you would like in the shop? You hate trying to combine this protein with that starch, or find yourself buying yet another dried thyme packet because you couldn't remember if you had one?

Planning a healthy meal takes work, and one of the most critical tasks is to shop for the ingredients. When you are trying to save money for food and have as many organic, healthy foods as possible on the table, the way you shop will be the first step in the path.

Here are some ideas for making your food trips quicker and better:

Roundup recipe. Food preparation calls for certain basic moves. You begin by thinking about what you want to do during the week. You can do this by selecting some meals that you know how to make with your heart, and also by choosing some recipes in blogs and magazines. Collect 6-8 recipes or food ideas and determine which to make for next week. Seek not to be too greedy and prepare an extravagant meal for a week. Accept your routine and seek to make fast and time- consuming dishes a good fit for your meals.

What's different about it? You will review the weekly circulars and flyers for salt products that suit your schedule once your meals are selected. When you have a budget, it can only help to pick things that are different. Now is the time to decide if there are any ingredients in your recipes that you can change. For example, if you want to make some turkey meatballs, but the ground chicken specials, switch the chicken.

Create a list and stick to it. This stage is very self-explaining, but cannot overestimate its value. Making a clear list of what you need from the supermarket helps the time you need to shop. It also helps you to counter the 'rolling belly syndrome' where you click the cart and look at everything on the shelf and unexpectedly drop a Nutella or ice cream into your cart if it isn't on your list. It also allows you to monitor it. At the time, it just looked like a good idea, right? Don't feel too bad, we all were there. Keep concentrating on the items on your agenda, while not having a lot of fun, will help save you!

Use the counter of the butcher or measure your meat. You can buy meat in precise quantities if you're fortunate enough to have access to the butcher shop or a good butcher counter in your local food shop. The problem that we always found in food stores is how the meat is sold. Families come in many sizes and requirements, but only two general sizes come with ground beef. When you buy a smaller box, your recipe can be short. When you buy one of these large packs of 5 pounds, then you have to split it into suitable sizes, or you can eventually cook it all.

In your shopping trip, meat is always the most significant expense. Buying bulk will save a lot of money, but only if you do it correctly. You will immediately portion and repackage your meat for freezer storage when you get it home. Usually, if you have purchased a fourth of beef from a cow, they divide it into the portions you choose. Wherever it came from, it's crucial not to allow your good intentions to buy your budget and portions in bulk sabotage. Some recipes call for pound meat; such as roasts or ground beef. Often you find that the only numbers you see are sums greater or smaller than what your shopping list needs. Use your discretion in that case and buy one that is either a little bigger or a little smaller than the amount you chose to purchase.

Vegetables and fruits. For the basis of a balanced diet, a variety of fruits and vegetables are essential to protect us from boredom. Many of us are fortunate enough to have access to a vast array of fresh produce all year long and can also find almost everything we want to eat.

Nevertheless, often fresh goods are costly. If in a Canadian February you have ever wanted red peppers, you know what that means. Why can all of your fresh vegetables be obtained without breaking? Often seek to replace an item for sale with what a recipe calls for. If it's expensive to get your hands on jicama, skip it and pick the same amount of pears. If the root of celery is $4 a pound (even!), move it on and take another form of the root. Recipes can still be adapted and changed; the budget can not be blown down by any ingredients.

Check it out if you live in a region with an Asian market. There are also goods at very low prices. Of course, the catch is that the product might have a spot here or a blur. These markets can indeed be a kind of establishment without frills, but the food is subject to the same food safety inspection rules as a typical food supplier. The costs are therefore much lower, and if you're not too picky when you arrange your limes in pyramids, you will undoubtedly pick up a bargain.

Pantry stuff. There are several things you often use, such as oils, stocks, and tomatoes. If non- perishable or durable items are on sale, take the opportunity to stock them. You will spend a little more on this outing, but it will take one thing off the next shopping list.

Often a recipe calls for an ingredient that you do not often store. For example, if you needed a half cup of pecans for a recipe, you'd put them on your shopping list. You could come to the store and find that they only sell them by the pack, which is much more than you want and need. If you don't want or have to buy a big volume, find it in bulk. Bulk stores are great places to buy items you like, for example, spices and unique ingredients. Need just a cup of quinoa? This won't be a problem in a bulk shop or in the bulk of your local grocery store.

If there's a fridge. As discussed above, a freezer is an ideal tool for bulk purchasers. When big sales rise or a lot of food is purchased at once, a freezer will help you ensure that nothing is lost. Knowing that there is some room in your freezer makes it easier to buy money-you won't struggle to reprogram your tiny regular freezer like a Tetris game later on.

If and when you hide things in the fridge, try to label it with the current date. We were all there; we hit the chest and took an anonymous foil packet and asked, "when did I freeze a ham?"

Get out of the supermarket. Who says you have to shop at the same place for your apples and salmon? Try to buy your greens from the following sources if you have access to them:

The demand for farmers:

The best things about a farmer's market are that many plants, such as purple cauliflowers or pet typical summer squash, you've never seen before can be found. Conventional grocery stores cannot always stock this specific commodity, so a farmer's market is the next best source of new foodstuffs. Moreover, the items you buy on the market were mostly harvested in the morning or the day before.

More than just work, a trip to the farmers' market. You will see the people behind your meal. The money you pay for squash is owns the person who grew it. There is some satisfaction that is difficult to duplicate in a shop.

Garden markets:

These markets are mostly seasonal mom and pop stores, which can also be nurseries for flowering. Often they're on a farm or a pick-your-own berry field, but they can be found in cities as well. Production is typically provided by local farmers but may include the same product in a supermarket. It's between a traditional grocery store and a farmer's market.

If you have time and energy to make, your own food-you should try it. If you have never before had a vegetable garden, you might want to stick to the easiest vegetables like tomatoes, cucumbers, and summer squash (zucchini). A packet of seeds from a non-GMO organic source will cost up to $1. It beats nothing to go outside to pick a tomato from your own garden.

CHAPTER FOUR: Meal plan in 3 weeks with recipes

We all heard the word 'superfood,' but you heard of sirtfoods? They're basically from the same generation. Perhaps even sirtfoods could be regarded as superfoods by themselves.

Both also serve similar structural functions in the body and provide more benefits as far as the internal workings of the body are concerned than the typical food.

Today we're going to think about meal preparation. Meals are among the most unforgettable elements of any camping trip, and you never hear the end when you have a disaster. This will show you how to avoid spending half the day in the kitchen and still eat a meal that knocks off your socks. Pre-planning and training are a perfect way to take more time to do what you've come through "Camping." later will share a recipe that provides a great way to prepare pasta. There are two meal preparation types, the method of ration, and the technique of recipes. This will focus on the process of resetting.

In a later problem, we will go through the ration method in detail. The recent approach is much more straightforward for a small group in a camp setting. Whether you have or need to be mobile, the rationing approach is preferable.

An efficient and fun way to plan your menu is to pick up all your favorite recipes and to make your daily menu, with no space or supply restrictions, focused on your scheduled activities. For starters, if you plan a walk, sandwiches will do the trick. You can buy more elaborate meals if you intend to live close to the place. You can be set once you hit the platform. You don't have to follow the tea line. Mix it up, be creative, and have fun.

When you have your menu, find out what items you will need and change your menu and/or equipment according to your room and weight needs. Otherwise, it can be a real challenge to create a menu. Our objective here is to have fun. This meal preparation approach is a simple way to figure out what resources you need without any estimation of your weight and height. There are several complicated formulas to use for meal planning, and these are important in certain situations such as backpacking and long journeys, but for the typical camping certainty, it is not necessary. When you forget or miss something, most campgrounds have a shop on-site or within a short drive. You can kick yourself because you have to spend twice what's worth, but you won't go hungry.

You can select from a vast amount of freshwater, high-quality snacks and fresh fruit, beef jerky, and granola in your menu. Keep away from stuff such as soda, chips, and cookies unless you want to lounge around the campsite and watch TV. The outdoor activity needs a lot of energy and calories to be burned. The easiest way to prepare healthy food is to use the ladder of the USDA Food Guide. Keep an appetite in mind as it is prepared.

Prepare as much as possible before planning and training. Use a cooler to preserve your peregrinations, including milk, condiments, and fresh vegetables. For all camp recipes, use powdered milk because it's handy to bring and easy to turn your recipe to fresh milk when you have it. Usually, for the first few days, use fresh milk, and then go to powdered milk after we run out. That's the plan, at least. Some children love to drink milk and always fit when we are fresh.

The positive thing about the meal menu planning strategy is that most home recipes can be adapted with very little effort into outdoor recipes. This next recipe is a great example of something just as tasty at home or online. Take note of pre-planning tips that make this a simple solution without losing taste.

Pasta Italiana Campsite.

- Italian Style: 1 28 oz.
- 1 tsp. of ground garlic.
- 4 Tbsp. of peanut or olive oil.
- Pasta 7 to 8 oz.
- 1 lb. of Italian sausage sliced to ½ inch.
- Parmesan Cheese.
- Salt and potatoes.

Cut sausages in front of your hand and store it in a zip lock bag.

Do Ahead Tip: Cook pasta in the box at home. Drain with cold water and clean. Place pasta and 2 tbsp. oil in a full pot. Throw in a zip lock bag and put in a cooler till required, until uniformly sealed.

Tip Ahead: Prepare multiple pasta dishes and simultaneously cook all the pasta. Hold every piece in a separate container. Using a permanent marker to write the name of the recipe for which each bag is intended.

Remove the correct pasta bag from the cooler before you make your meal and let it hit room temperature.

Heat 2 tablespoons of oil in a medium-high big bowl. Remove sausage and brown until evenly fried. Drain the fat; add the crushed tomatoes, and the garlic powder. Constantly stir and bring to a boil, reducing heat to medium. Simmer for about 5 to 10 minutes until thickened. Remove heat and add pasta. Remove. Mix well. Mix well. When the pulp is too small to add, all the ingredients can be combined in a large pot. The sauce 's heat will heat up the pasta. Serve with parmesan cheese and apply salt and pepper to compare.

LOW BUDGET MEAL PLANNING

How much money your family earns hard goes to food? 200 dollars a week? 150 dollars?

Believe it or not, it is possible (although difficult) to spend as little as $75 a week on a family of five or six. But raising the food charge to those lower numbers means that you will have to reconsider how your family eats.

For busy families today, the nearby driveway restaurant is always easier to swing, rather than having time and energy to prepare a new meal every night. Quick food is not only an expensive choice for your children; it is not just the healthiest way to eat regularly.

You aren't alone if this defines your dinnertime problem. For several fast and easy meals, keep the right ingredients.

Cook several of your meals ahead for quick preparation later in the week in the freezer. To create a stockpile of frozen assets quickly, you can simply repeat and replicate recipes every now and then as you cook regularly during the week. When placed in the freezer, all you need to do is heat a meal and prepare a side dish or salad for one of the all-too-frequent busy nights without any time to cook. By preparing in advance, you can also save money by purchasing bulk ingredients and making use of market sales.

Offer breakfast for dinner sometimes. Even when cooked in a big way, breakfast has been one of the cheapest food to cook. In many busy homes, relatives rarely have time to have a large breakfast of pancakes, eggs, and bacon in the morning, so having a meal such as that for dinner sometimes is a very special treat. Omelettes always make a good choice for dinner.

SIMPLIFYING FOOD PREPARATION

You can use your residues for lunches brought from home instead of buying lunch every day by planning and cooking larger meals at the diner.

Take one night a week for your children to feed for the entire family. It can be as easy as opening a soup can and preparing sandwiches of grilled cheese.

Slow cookers are perfect for fast cooking-just put the ingredients into the hook early in the morning and have dinner when you get home.

AHEAD PLANNING

Also, if you do not feel that cooking for a whole month will be of interest to you or your family, it may potentially simplify preparing meals for the month in advance and also save money.

Set the food and gas budget first, and then make the menus and food list appropriate for the budget-not the reverse. Decide what you can afford, and don't get it out. You would be surprised if you knew that you could only spend "this lot and nothing more" in the store.

Take a few minutes to plan a monthly menu and write down everything you need for every meal in the building. Look into the freezer and the cabinets to see what you have. So look at your calendar to see what the monthly things are like —note any birthday party, an evening when everyone leaves the house for a quick meal, occasions when people eat at home, or other events that could affect your meal plans for the month.

Then take a look at your local food shops' flyers. Plan your food for what's on offer and what you already have on hand to save the most money. When you plan to shop every week, prepare all your weekly food lists in advance of the month (write the whole month of shopping lists in a single day, so all you need to do when it's time to shop).

Write your meal schedule down on a blank calendar page and hang it on an easily accessible spot (fridge, family newsletter board). It took time to draw up the menu and food lists, but it saves more time every day and creates a lot less tension when you decide what to eat that night.

BUYING FOOD CO-OPS

Make sure to look for grocery buying co-ops in your local areas. Some have low subscription fees, which you can recover easily from substantial discounts on other frequently purchased products. Natural food companies are common and are an excellent way of buying organic fruit and vegetables, whole grains, and other expensive products at competitive prices.

Many societies offer a food sharing system known as Sharing. For a total cost of $14 and 2 hours of community, service members will be given a $35-$40 food package. Community service may be as easy as supporting an elderly neighbor or volunteering at your nursery or Sunday school. The shares also sell meatless shares and normal foodstuffs.

You can also begin your own small, unofficial bulk food shopping with a group of friends or neighbors. You can then divide the item into family quantities and split the cost by buying products such as food, sugar, wheat cream, oats, etc., in big bulk cartons (50 pounds).

Many people from their local club store purchase large amounts of products. Although most of the products in these stores can be purchased at big discounts, you can still shop here in contrast. Sometimes you will find that sales in your local food shop are actually cheaper per pound or item than in the big warehouse stores. Bring a machine always with you to make sure you get the best price per package.

Remember, make sure you purchase only certain things in the quantity that you are confident you need before they go wrong. Toilet paper storage is a smart idea because it is one of the things that you know that you will eventually need. It might not be a good idea to store bananas on sale, as they spoil easily unless you intend to bake with them or freeze banana pulp later on.

Sirtfood vs superfood

Sirtfoods Are Also Syrtuins

Sirtfoods help to maintain low inflammation, encourage metabolism, loss of weight, immunity, and healthy aging.

What is the diet? What is the diet?

The miracle argument is that if you observe your Sirtfood diet carefully, you will lose 7 pounds in 7 days. But don't worry – we aren't big fans of extreme claims fad diets.

The foundation is essential, and we personally think the underlying nutritional goal is very sustainable, so listen to us! If we're not conscious yet, there's chocolate, and there's wine.

The first week has a reasonable clear food schedule for implementing. Do you recall that promise? Okay, on your side, it comes with a little effort.

For first, it sounds a little restricting and 'cleansing,' but it's getting better. Each day, you'll want about 1,000 calories, including three glasses of green juice and one meal rich in sirt food.

During the second week, you can increase your calorie intake to 1.500 calories a day, including two green juices and two sirtfood-rich meals.

Following this, there is no real rhyme or justification for your Sirtfood diet, so we like it! The idea is simply to have as much sirtfood as possible in your diet to activate sirtuins that will keep our cells healthy and vibrant, avoid inflammation, disease, and excess weight.

Overall, we agree that this is a positive solution to include more whole foods rich in vitamins and minerals and greens in the diet.

In general, the long-term agenda requires three sirtfood-rich foods a day and one green juice. In the following weeks after the presentation, you can expect a gradual loss of weight at a safe pace.

Why do we want to die in the sirtfood?

In view of the limits on calories, you may wonder why we put our stock in our Sirtfood Diet. Despite the "rapid weight loss" and lose guidelines, though, we think it goes beyond the fad diet mindset.

First, the transition takes place in steps, so that the 1000 days of calories do not last long. If you've ever tried out the diet, you probably know it leads only to hunger!

Our 9-week Healthy Body Recipe menu includes many of the same foods we use. In our reset period, we remove wine and chocolate, but re-introduce these foods, as we agree that they have antioxidants and the potential to restore balance to the diet.

Who doesn't enjoy life's more beautiful things? We love the sirtfood diet that helps you to enjoy some excellent health benefits.

This 'diet' is used to keep the immune system more energetic and healthier over time. Sirtfoods serve a higher purpose in the body, and over and above weight loss. That said, it provides a very affordable lifelong wellness network.

The immune system is close to our general well-being, and it is necessary to provide the body with the resources that our cells need to stay healthy and to reduce inflammation caused by illness.

In all, the Sirtfood Diet is about putting the most abundant foods in your daily diet with vitamins and minerals multiple times daily. It's a basic idea with a straightforward formula and substantial advantages.

SuperFoods: Just a Title

You've already learned a lot of "superfoods" lately. Announcements will allow you to buy chlorella, blue-green algae dubbed "Nature 's Great Superfood." Information about superfoods from the reputable and unreputable sources is available.

People like WebMD and the respected Center for Public Interest Science (CSPI) are tapping into the craze. We give information on "Superfoods' everyone wants" and the "10 Superfoods for improved health!" The numerous (and questionable) remedies and elixirs make unrealizable claims on the not-so-reputable hand. We offer quick and easy delivery of superfoods, without even eating food.

But what about these superfoods? So what would you do with all the superfood hype?

SUPERFOOD AND SIRTFOOD

The idea of "super-foods" often begins with an interest in certain foods found in only a few particular cultures or regions of the world. Soy foods are an example of one of the first 'superfoods.' In the far East Asian countries such as Japan and Korea, traditional soy foods like tofu, tempeh, and miso were initially consumed. Soy has been destroyed in these areas for thousands of years.

Such regions and countries still experience some of the lowest chronic disease rates in the world. Cardiovascular levels, obesity, diabetes, a stroke, high blood pressure, and much more are a fraction of what they are in the US and other Western countries.

Soy food is a sharp contrast in diet between Asia and many countries in the West. This led people to believe that soy products were 'extra' or 'good' in terms of disease prevention. It may seem to be a reasonable inference. Many Asian cultures eat soy. Most Asian societies have deficient levels of disease. Soy foods must also avoid illness.

Urban Asian soy products can be used in a balanced diet. These foods do indeed produce plant nutrients in abundance. And scientific evidence supports the protective disease properties of whole soy foods.

However, it is not accurate that the superior health and longevity observed in many Asian countries is soy and soy alone. There are so many variations between Asian and western cultures, dietary and otherwise. It would be a mistake to smash low disease rates into soy apart.

Asians are typically thinner. Sometimes they get more exercise, sleep, and less fat in their diet than Americans. We will have more robust social and family networks and fewer burdens in their lives. They eat fewer foods and more vegetables. They consume plants that in western cultures like algae are never or rarely eaten. All this (and more) undoubtedly leads to lower levels of disease in many parts of Asia.

All this points to something obvious that we sometimes forget about superfoods in our excitement: No food is an answer to good health. In fact, many other nutritional factors contribute to good health. The bottom line is that there are really no superfoods. Then, we will try to find out what constitutes a superdiet.

In your diet, but the "Super."

One of many in the case of soy is a superfood. The items on the top of the "superfood" list, presumably have similar tales. Everybody has an example of their favorite superfood from acai (ah-sigh-ee) and goji berries through to matcha root and green tea. They should point to the food and superior health that the society that consumes it has to bring. It is proven to be "super" or very unique.

However, if you look a little more deeply, you'll find that both of these cultures' diet is essential to the positive health benefits. As part of the Mediterranean diet, olive oil is widely marketed as a path to good health. But besides olive oil, you'll find some nuts, fish, seeds, fruits, vegetables, lower body weights, moderated red wines, less red meat, etc.

In short, we need to concentrate on consuming a healthy diet rather than the traditional superfood. What's the feel of a superfood? Think plants. Remember plants. Science primarily supports the fact that herbal food is essential to good health and lower disease levels. Plant-based doesn't have to mean vegetarian, but it's all right if you choose. Plant-based basically means that most of your calories come from unrefined and low-processed foods.

Your site preparation

Starting with your plate is the best way to use nutrition to reduce your own risk of diseases, including cancer and heart disease.

Divide a traditional round plate into four pie-shaped wedges in your head. There should be three out of these four wedges of vegetables (most considerable portions), fruit (a little less than veggies), and whole grains (no more than one serving per meal or snack). Lean protein, including chicken, fish, breasts, or lean beef, can be included in the final wedge.

You may want to focus on variety in addition to these steps. Again, note that there is no "strong enough" food to provide a complete mix of minerals, vitamins, and phytonutrients required for good health. Instead, you want to use the healing power of as many whole plant foods as possible.

Eat foods, blue, green, red, yellow, purple, and orange. Kale, chard, and kiwi (green); pines, maize, and banana (yellow); peppers, strawberries, beans, raspberries, and tomatoes (red); pancakes, prunes, blueberries, and raisins (purple); and carrots, grapes, and sweet potatoes and melon (orange). These are just a handful of the hundreds of fun foods you need to eat a healthy diet.

We all understand that to get healthy and stay healthy, what you put into your body and on your plate at every meal is one of the best ways to start. Nutrient-rich foods are natural sources of vitamins and disease-free things for your body. Best of all, at any age, you will begin to enjoy these top superfoods!

By twenty-something...

Make sure you do whatever you can to develop your bone mass because this is your last chance. According to government figures, more than 50 % of women in their 20s are not getting the calcium they need every day (1000 mg). Some of us get around half of it. Afterward, eating well and exercising will help to preserve your bone mass in these years.

A cup of plain unfitted yogurt, one cup of fortified soy milk or orange juice, a cup of fat-free milk, or an amount of cheddar cheese are the primary sources of calcium build-up.

Folate is another essential nutrient at this age, and you should be mindful of how much you are receiving when you decide to get pregnant. Up to 70 percent (including *spina bifida*) of neural tube defects can be avoided if women get the right amount of this essential vitamin. Also, if you just "push" 400 mcg every day and get up to 600 mcg while you are pregnant.

You'll want your folate as an extra tool for better absorption and seek out natural sources such as 100 percent folic acid daily value cereals (400 mcg), four spears of asparagus, 1 ounce of raw spinach or a slice of whole-wheat bread.

By thirty-something...

Iron is a phenomenal exhaustion fighter, which is essential to balancing family, work, and relationships in the time of your life. Most women in this age group don't eat a lot of meat, so experts don't prescribe 18 mg of iron. Animal protein is the best kind of metal in your body, and however, if you pair with foods loaded with vitamin C, such as strawberries or red peppers, plant food will give you more.

Cup fortified cereal (18 mc of iron), half-cup white beans, a half-cup of cooked spinach, 3 ounces of beef, or chicken are the highest sources of your iron sources.

The 30s also provide an excellent time to help the heart by adding omega-3 fats, as your regular consumption of them can reduce your risk of heart disease by lowering triglycerides. You would want to eat at least two portions of fish each week (choose low mercury varieties). Omega-3 seafood sources are best for brain health.

Three ounces of salmon, halibut, flounder, shrimp, or canned light tuna are the best options for these safe heart omega-3.

For forty-something...

Fiber is your companion in the 1940s, allowing you to sleep better and eat less. Around this age, your metabolism is slowing down, and your muscle mass is slowing down, thus raising the calories you need every day by about 100. Fiber also maintains constipation (more frequently when you get older) while also reducing cholesterol. We need 25 grams every day, but most women get much less.

Get enough half cup of 100% bran, half a cup of black boar, half a cup of pear, half a cup of raspberries, an ounce, or half a cup of whole-wheat pasta.

At this age, potassium is another good nutrient. This is the time of life when blood pressure can start to shrink, but if you do something, you can avoid medications. Having ample potassium doesn't reduce the high blood pressure; it also works well against the effects of sodium rise in blood pressure. It may cause even every bone loss. Touch the 4,700 mg a day to get your body benefits.

Choose plenty of a medium sweet potato or cabbage, a medium banana, 3 oz of pork, a cup of fat, free milk, or a half cup of cooked lentils.

Good science is now available to support food rich in antioxidants that could save you from cognitive decline (including Alzheimer's and dementia). You 're going to want the most antioxidant materi

al you can, so try five portions of fruit and vegetables every day.

A cup of berries, half cup of drizzled prunes, a Granny Smith apple, a cup of red raisins- vegetables include medium-russet pulp, a cup of

artichoke hearts, half cup of broccoli or a half cup of raw red col-
would be the most effective antioxidant bets.

By fifty-something...

Now is the time for vitamin D to really help; every cell in your body
needs this nutrient to function. This may explain why it is related to
so many health benefits, from lowering cancer risk to depression
defense. You want to try out the minimum 400 IU, but people at this
age make about 30% less from simple exposure to the sun, so that
even more important is what you get from diet.

The best bets on vitamin D include three ounces of light tuna, one cup
of milk/juice enhanced by D or one egg. Most multivitamins give you
400IUs a day, but you may want to add 1,000 IU of vitamin D a day.
Another significant nutrient, B12, will help you stay healthy, but the
majority of people over 50 will not generate enough stomach acid for
the food we are consuming to absorb the vitamin. This is concerning
as this vitamin is essential for the development of red blood cells and
is used in the brain. Deficient B12 levels can lead to an increase in
homocysteine associated with cardiac disease. If you are concerned,
your doctor can check your B12 levels.

There is an age in which you will be better off getting the B12 also
because you can handle it faster and more reliably. You may need a
multivitamin or a bowl of fortified cereal (100% DV B12). 2.5mcg
every day is what you're going to shoot for. A cup of this fortified
cereal, three oz. of beef, a cup of yogurt or a cup of milk are some

essential sources of B12.

Sirtdiet and exercises

Live a balanced lifestyle is one of the main factors to delay the aging process. It involves eating whole foods, exercising every day, not smoking, and reducing alcohol intake. Keeping your body safe would also protect you against the danger of type 2 diabetes, high blood pressure, and cardiovascular diseases.

When telling patients to keep up with the food they consume to keep them looking and feeling beautiful, the same question always comes down to me: 'What are the best ingredients you have to prepare in order to remain healthy?' Whether you eat is not as important as how much food has been refined. The expression "full food" is nowadays a household word, but what does it mean?

Whole food implies to foods that are minimally processed and graded as rich in nutrients. This contains vitamins, antioxidants phytonutrients, minerals, starch, fatty acids of omega-3, calcium, and anti-inflammatory substances; this provides every protection that nature has to offer. The best thing about whole foods is that all these essential nutrients produce a minimal amount of calories.

On the other hand, refined, dried, and fast foods are known as nutrient deficient because of the limited amount of nutrients in contrast to a large number of calories they produce. It is not surprising that a healthy combination of whole foods is recommended for weight control and optimum health, mainly when organically grown and cooked correctly.

The best diet is based on whole foods with minimal processing regardless of the number of grams of grains, protein, or fat it includes. Let's look at some of the foods recognized for all their nutritional benefits.

Nuts, Beans, Beans, Oh My!!!!!

Many excellent foods are pure, natural and unprocessed, and almost always are right, whether they are used as additives to recipes, snacks, or main meal additives. Nuts, bananas, beans, vegetables, and onions belong to the list of favorites, which is why.

It has been shown that eating nuts minimize the risk of heart disease. Beer is low in calories, high in fiber, and full of antioxidants that improve the memory and help fight cancer. Beer does have molecules that can prevent the development of tumors.

Beans of all kinds, in particular lentils, are rich in fiber and basically unfit and make a dish that is similar to the protein content of red meals or dairies in combination with whole grains or pasta. To every dish, add beans like marine, pinto, or black beans, and increase the nutritional value. In the 1999 epidemiological report, which monitored 13,000 male subjects over 25 years, more legumes were eaten with an 82% reduction in the risk of death due to cardiovascular disease.

There are almost no losers when it comes to vegetables. Some of them stand out while others take their back seats based on their planning or consumption. Too many you put on your salads or herbs that increase the calories and offset the excellent gain.

For starters, potatoes are often lousy rap because they are typically associated with French fries filled with saturated fat. It's a self-sufficient veggie filled with vitamins B6 and vitamins C, fiber, potassium, and many other poly nutrients and is separated from a baked potato by your butter, sour cream, and bacon.

The emphasis is on chicken, Brussels sprouts, broccoli, and kale filled with chemicals called dolphins to help reduce the cancer risk. Apples are undoubtedly one of the fruit kingdom's superstars as they are filled with mineral, fiber, and phytochemicals that have proven anti-cancer properties.

Without the *Alliaceae* family of plants, what would be onions, meal, garlic, and shallots? In addition to the phytochemical compounds, they provide you with a punch that speeds up the reduction of carcinogenesis in your body.

A variety of studies have shown that garlic can decrease the risk of heart disease, while the onion is known for its positive effect on some forms of cancer.

Do not forget teas, mainly green, which have long been promoted as the safest foods in the world because they are filled with plant chemicals known as catechins to combat cancer and inflammation.

Cook your heart to safety

It is essential to understand not only why whole foods are right for you, but also why you need to learn the best way to cook them to optimize your health benefits. Choose the fat types that decrease cholesterol content and use a cooking method that retain all the nutrients of the food you prepare, such as steaming, broiling, baking, microwaving, roasting, or grilling.

Natural eating is also the safest way to get the most significant number of vitamins and minerals for vegetables. The next best thing is to microwave or steam instead of boiling your veggie 's future. When sautéing, make sure to use olive oil instead of butter to reduce your consumption of fat.

Search for recipes that give flavor rather than fat to use herbs and spices. Squeezing lemon on steamed vegetables, grilled fish, rice, or pasta will accomplish this. Spice stuff with onion and garlic or using chicken or pork BBQ sauce.

The right variety of poultry, beef, or pork will help hold the objective of your cholesterol.

- Beef – Choose lean cuttings such as small, sirloin and flank steak, bait, rib, chuck or rump, bone, porter or cubed steak

- Poultry-choose not dark (white is less fat), without skin and white.

- Pork-ham, pork loin, Canadian bacon, far middle chops are the lean styles

Consider products that are made of non-fat or low-fat milk while attempting to minimize saturated fat.

A balanced diet does not consist of bland, tasty, boring foods. You can make your meals even more enjoyable than before by following some simple guidelines: Eat organic, unprocessed foods, saturated fats, and cook wisely. Perhaps you're just going to lose weight and look fantastic! How could it be better than that now?

SUPPLEMENT FOOD AND EXERCISE

Adding weight loss to a certain amount of exercise and food preparation, and your mealtime routine will make an obese person a weight-burning champion!

Weight loss and weight consuming supplement

Even like your body needs pure water, you'd accept that you need self-love, the warmth of the sun and clean air! Knowing that the number of people who don't love their bodies is fantastic!

We tend to like and enjoy their junk food only because it has an effect on their taste buds. Junk- food establishments have developed and use enticing marketing tactics vigorously. Young children seem to be a strategy that businesses in Junk Food use very frequently!

Obesity or extra weight is caused by storing fat and not consuming waste. Everybody wants fat in their everyday diet, what happens with a weight loss supplement is that fat burning kicks in! The excess fat thus is a non-event!

Besides the distinct requirements of the body, as mentioned earlier, the body requires food, protein, carbon, and other fats. Your hope also is that these products provide the vitamins and minerals that your body needs to function efficiently and avoid disease. You can hope, but it is easier to use other natural fat loss supplements to help in the process of fat burning.

Avoiding the three meals a day system you have cultivated will help your body process the food you eat! You do this by choosing smaller foods and more. When you lock in meals, you can primarily be sure that your body has not digested the meal before and that it does as it has been told it stores it!

You want to make sure your body removes extra fat and keeps your body healthy. A weight-loss replacement system includes the main elements, some exercise and food intake in the lower glycemic index. Right breaks in meals are just as significant.

Fat loss aid and glycemic index

The Glycemic Index is a calculation of the blood sugar effect of carbohydrates. Low G I levels are slow to break down because glucose escapes gradually into your bloodstream. Carbs that quickly break down have a high level of G I.

Unfortunately, there is no future in junk foods for obese and overweight people since they are always high on the Glycemic Index. High G-I food consumption can be a significant reason for the enormous rise in illness, disability, and death for hundreds of millions of people. Obesity is a big concern worldwide.

In September 2008, Low Glycemic Index information from the Canadian Diabetes Assn showed that G I foods can help:

- Reduce your level of blood sugar.

- Lower the risk of diabetes type 2.

- Limit the cholesterol.

- Reduce the risk of heart disease.

- Check your appetite.

Fat loss supplements mean any movement

Natural fat loss minerals combined with low glycemic index food can help you lose fat and improve your energy levels. But by starting daily exercises, you can further enhance your strength. The positive news is that if you feel more motivated, the tasks will be more straightforward. It is where you 'tight your belt' seriously.

A guy recently told me that he used to leave the bus a stop early six months ago and walk the rest of the way to work or home. He gets off the three stops soon now! You should make time for your own well-being in different ways. Some kind of workout – just do it! For heart safety and physical activity, you must keep your blood flowing for muscle tone and strength. As the weight goes off and you can feel healthier inside and outside with a new fat lossplan! Fat Loss Results

Complement

To be useful in a fat loss supplement, you just don't want to be excessive in opioids, caffeine, or smoking tobacco. Emotional problems also do not help to lose weight. Such issues will make your health problems worse and find ways to eradicate them one by one will allow you to lead a healthier life.

People who want to lose weight sometimes forget basic things like drinking a glass of water if you're hungry. You should actually drink eight glasses of water every day. You have to shape your body to realize that there is no water shortage. Because your body starts retaining water (fluid retention), if you do not drink enough water, one thing that people also struggle to do is spend 10-15 minutes enjoying sunshine every day. We take the sunlight vitamin D, which is an essential element since there are no other components.

If you want to lose weight and improve health, it's better to have excellent support! The safest place to get this kind of help is at home. Community interest in healthy eating is half the battle. You are taking it with both hands if it is open. Naturally, this helps to clear all those delicacies from the pantry. Make sure you have a good breakfast, and fruit snacks are available at work and between meals. Watch sizes of meals, and you want to burn them, not store them!

Overweight people are not responsible for their own bodies. That's why they're too heavy! By combining extra fat loss minerals, lower glycemic foods, and physical activity, you can take over your body.

CONCLUSION

Sirtfood food intake is the new way of quickly changing weight without any radical diet by activating the same 'skinny gene' pathways usually only caused by exercise and fasting. Some foods contain chemicals known as polyphenols that place mild stress on our cells and turn on genes that replicate the effects of fasting and exercise. The sirtuin pathways which affect metabolism, aging, and the mood are triggered by foods rich in polyphenols, including kale, dark chocolate, and red wine. A diet rich in this sirtfood begins to lose weight, while maintaining optimal health, without sacrificing muscle.

Fill your diet with healthy sirtfoods for effective and sustained weight loss, extraordinary energy, and glistening health. Switch on the fat-burning power of your body, overload weight loss, and help prevent disease by using this easy-to-follow diet developed by nutritional experts who have demonstrated the impact of sirtfood. Dark chocolate, coffee, and kale – these are all foods, which activate the so-called "skinny gene" tracks in the body and activate sirtuins. The Sirtfood Diet provides you with a simple and balanced diet, tasty easy to make recipes, and an extended performance maintenance plan. The Sirtfood Diet is an inclusion diet without exclusion, and sirt food is readily available and affordable. This is a diet that encourages you to take your knife and bifurcate and enjoy savory food while watching health benefits and weight loss.

There is growing evidence that sirtuin activators can have a range of health benefits as well as muscle building and appetite suppression. These include better memory, helping the body control blood sugar levels more effectively, and cleansing the damage from free radical molecules that can build up in cells, cancer, and other diseases.

Substantial observational evidence is present for the positive effects of the consumption of foods and beverages rich in sirtuin activators, which minimize the risk of chronic disorders. A sirtfood diet is especially suited as an anti-aging diet.

While the entire plant kingdom has sirtuin activators, only some fruits and vegetables have adequate amounts as a sirtfood. For starters, green tea, cacao powder, Indian turmeric spice, onions, kale, and parsley.

In the supermarkets, many of the fruit and vegetables such as tomatoes, avocados, bananas, cabbage, kiwi, carrots, and cucumber are generally tiny in sirtuin activators. This doesn't mean they 're not worth eating, though, because they offer many other advantages.

The beauty of a sirtfood-packed diet is that it is much more flexible than other diets. You could just eat a few sirtfoods healthily. Or you could focus on them. The 5:2 diet could enable more calories in low-calorie days by adding sirtfood.

A notable finding from one Sirtfood diet study is that the participants lost considerable weight without reducing muscle. Yes, it was normal for participants to gain muscle, which resulted in a more refined and toned look. That's the beauty of sirtfoods: fat burning is enabled, but also muscle development, repairs, and maintenance are encouraged. It is in direct contrast to other diets, where weight loss usually comes from both fat and muscle, which slows down the process of muscle loss and makes it more challenging to return to weight.

CPSIA information can be obtained
at www.ICGtesting.com
Printed in the USA
LVHW082057091220
673699LV00001B/2

9 781801 256421